D1541581

Medicine Under Capitalism

Medicine Under Capitalism

Vicente Navarro
The Johns Hopkins University

PRODIST
NEW YORK

First published in the United States by
PRODIST
a division of
Neale Watson Academic Publications, Inc.
156 Fifth Avenue, New York 10010

Second printing 1977

Contents

Since it is not for us to create a plan for the future that will hold for all time, all the more surely what we contemporaries have to do is the uncompromising critical evaluation of all that exists, uncompromising in the sense that our criticism fears neither its own results nor the conflict with the powers that be.

Karl Marx, letter to Arnold Ruge, 1844.

Introduction

The essays in this collection are aimed at challenging the prevailing ideologies in the social sciences in general, and their application in the analysis and explanation of the Western system of medicine in particular. Originally published at different times and in different forums, these essays have in some cases been updated and in others pruned, with the intention of keeping them relevant and, although interrelated, distinct. Diverse in subject matter and even in tone, they nonetheless share an underlying purpose of questioning prevalent explanations of health and medicine and of presenting alternative ones.

It is my belief that the overwhelming influence—amounting to dominance—of functionalism in the social sciences in the Western world determines a focus of analysis and methods of inquiry that are not only limited and limiting, but often serve to obfuscate rather than to clarify our realities. It is a characteristic of these analyses, for example, that they focus on the parts, supposedly in order to lead later to the comprehension of the whole, i.e. they study the components of society prior to studying society itself. Indeed, it is assumed that after the cool, analytical look at the parts, one can later develop a theoretical model of the whole society, however abstract that model, like the Parsonian one, may be. And this approach has been particularly marked in the analysis of medicine. In that respect, most analyses in the social science of the house of medicine—in their conservative, liberal, and sometimes even radical versions—have focused on forces and actors *within* medicine, forces and actors that have been and continue to be considered the main determinants of events in that sector. But, as the saying goes, asking the right questions is more than half of getting the right answers, and asking the wrong questions assures never getting the right answers. And to focus on forces and actors within medicine in order to understand its ideology, composition, functions, distribution, production, or whatever, is to ask the wrong questions and therefore cannot lead to the right answers. Such an approach assumes that the part (medicine) is autonomous from the whole (society), an assumption that I question and with which I disagree. To the contrary, and as I show in the essays in this volume, the system of medicine is determined primarily—although not exclusively—by the same forces that determine the overall social formation, society. In other words, I consider medicine to be the dialectical result of forces that exist both outside and within medicine. And in a gradient of influence, the former ranks higher than the latter. This, then, leads to the need to understand the whole of our social reality and the forces that determine it.

But this analysis of the forces that determine the shape and nature of our societies is severely hindered by the present division of labor in the social sciences, where the investigation of our realities is parceled out among several closely knitted disciplinary kingdoms, i.e. economics, sociology, anthropology, political science, and others. Indeed, the disciplinary approach in the social sciences leads to a situation where the understanding of our realities is intrinsically and unavoidably fragmented, preventing the comprehension of both the totality and of the underlying determinants of that totality. As a result of this division of labor in the social sciences, political science, for example, does not deal with the basic economic forces, while conversely, economy neglects and obscures the social class relations, and so on and so forth. Indeed, while the Hegelian dictum that "the truth is the whole" continues with an undiminished validity, the disciplinary approach prevalent in today's social sciences perpetuates the one-sided tunnel vision that impedes our vision of the totality. And to the same degree that the whole is always more than the sum of its parts, the explanation of our reality and its different components, including medicine, is more—far more—than the mere aggregate of its sociological, economic, political, psychological, and other explanations. Actually, it is not so much a question of *more,* but rather a question of *different.* And by this I mean that the comprehension of our societies and their medical realities requires not a unidisciplinary or an aggregate (i. e. multidisciplinary) approach, but an altogether different approach, in which the subject of analysis—in this case, medicine—is viewed as part of the larger social formation—society—of which it is a component, analyzing the dialectical relationships between that part and the whole.

This is the approach I use in these essays. In that respect, I am counterposing Marxism—the method of social analysis used here—to the methods traditionally used and prevalent in the various disciplines in social science. In contrast with prevalent patterns of orthodoxy, for example, I do not use a disciplinary analysis of the components of society in order to later understand society; but rather, and as the Marxist method does, I focus first on the analysis of the entire social system, and then use the understanding of the whole as the necessary basis for the analysis and understanding of the parts. In other words, I try to show how medicine—the part—is determined by the same forces that determine society—the whole. And by society, I mean, in the Marxist sense, the social arrangements determined in the final analysis by a specific combination of social forces and relations of production.[1] In the following essays, I identify that specific combination, existent in most of the Western world studied in this volume, as capitalism, thus explaining the title selected for this volume—*Medicine Under Capitalism.*

Let me add here that I am aware, of course, of the mythology prevalent in large sectors of the social sciences that we have transcended paradigms such as capitalism, and instead we have "mixed economies" or "post-industrial societies" in the world of development, or "third world countries" in the world of underdevelopment. In many of the essays in this volume, I challenge this assumption. My postulate is that, while changes of a most substantial nature in the Western world have indeed occurred, they have not altered the fundamental characteristics and contradictions of capitalism, there for all to see. In spite of this, the paradigms of capitalism, imperialism, social class, class struggle and others used in Marxist theory, are usually dismissed, both in the bourgeois press and academia, as irrelevant and as subjects of concern only to incorrigible ideologues who are supposedly oblivious to the passage of time. Those terms are thus quickly cast into exile in a note of introduction; and when used, they are generally placed between quotation marks, as if to alert the reader that they are subjects of suspicion. In that respect, it is interesting to note that in prevalent discourse, Marxism is presented as an *ideology,* while social sciences are presented as *science.* That dichotomous interpretation flows from the understanding of the task of the social sciences as one of collecting information and evidence which can be ascertained independently of any political position or value judgment.

Indeed, in the social sciences, the study of society and its component parts is assumed to be based on the simple accumulation of facts, from which theories are then, and only then, deduced. In this way, theories come to be regarded as hovering above the *terra firma* of established fact and empirically-tested hypotheses. The main assumption behind that dichotomy—an engagingly naive one at that—is that a realm of facts exists independent of the theories which establish their meaning. In other words, it is assumed that facts are on the one side, and theory on the other. But, contrary to that assumption, I do not believe in such a dichotomy. As I attempt to show in many of these essays, theory already exists in the genesis, choice and interpretation of facts. In that respect, one is not built upon the other. The one is in the other. There is, thus, no

[1]Marx, K. *Grundrisse.* Penguin, Middlesex, 1973.

possibility of having a "value free" social science. What usually passes as such is merely the analysis of reality, taking *as given* the already existent values implied in both the facts and their interpretation. Not surprisingly, such "value free" analysis has been defined as "status quo" social science.[2] In summary, then, all social analysis, however dispassionate or adorned with elegant statistical presentation, or no matter how pompous the sociologese in which it is couched, is value-laden. And all social sciences are ideologies in disguise. By analyzing the prevalent interpretations of medicine in most disciplinary areas of social science, these essays aim to prove it.

Themes of the Volume

The essays presented here were written in particular cultural and political settings. In this volume, however, they have been arranged thematically, grouped into four parts. The first part includes four articles showing how the same political and economic forces that determine the nature of capitalism and imperialism also determine the underdevelopment of health and health resources. The first essay postulates that the present maldistribution of human health resources in Latin America is brought about by the same determinants that cause the general underdevelopment of most of that continent. There, I indicate that, contrary to the Parsonian and Rostowian theories of development prevalent in the corridors of power and the academic circles of developed countries (as well as in the leading circles of developing countries and in the international agencies), underdevelopment and the uneven distribution of resources inside and outside the health sector are not due to either (a) the absence of cultural and technologic diffusion from developed to developing countries, (b) the scarcity of capital in poor nations, or (c) the presence of dual economies in underdeveloped countries, i.e. the urban-entrepreneurial economy and the rural primitive economy. To the contrary, underdevelopment and the concomitant maldistribution of resources are caused precisely because of the existence of the assumed "conditions" of development, i.e. (a) the cultural, technologic, and economic dependency of developing countries, and (b) economic and political control of resources by specific interests and social groups—the national lumpenbourgeoisie and its foreign coun-

[2]Therborn, G. *Science, Class and Society. On the Formation of Sociology and Historical Materialism.* New Left Books, London, 1976.

terparts. Moreover, these two factors bring about the so-called "dual economies" found in these countries.

Within this scenario, it is important to analyze the experience of Chile—before, during and after Allende's administration—and this is the subject of the second essay. Chile shows that the same classes and groups whose behavior—determined by the internal logic of capitalism and imperialism—explains the sickness of underdevelopment, also explains the underdevelopment of health and health resources. The latter cannot be resolved within the parameters of the former. Both are determined by an economic and political system where the many control and own very little, and the few control and own quite a lot. In this situation resides the cause of the underdevelopment of health.

A similar, although not identical, causation appears in developed capitalist countries. The underdevelopment of health of large parts of rural America, and the lack of protection at the working place of the majority of working class America, presented in essays three and four, is due not to prevalent lifestyles—as the behavioral theorists indicate— but rather to the dramatic maldistribution of economic and political power in our society, with the absence of control by the majority of the U.S. population—the working and lower-middle classes—over the work process with which they are involved, the economic wealth that they produce, and the political institutions that they pay for. The production of goods and wealth, as well as the political institutions of the U.S., are dominated by a minority of our population—the corporate and upper-middle class. This pattern of dominance is determined not by a conspiracy—and I am not a conspiratorial theorist—but by the internal logic of capitalism that explains that underdevelopment of health and of health services.

Within this scenario, presented in Part I, medicine is supposed to take care of and, if possible, solve the underdevelopment of health. But according to a growing body of theorists—one of them being Ivan Illich— medicine, controlled by the medical profession, is seriously handicapped in this function, as a result of its industrialization and technologicalization. And, because of this, medicine has become a source of harm and oppression rather than a vehicle of relief and liberation. This explanation of medicine is part and parcel of the ideology of industrialism, which explains the nature and form of our societies as determined by the all-pervasive process of industrialization that invades all spheres of individual and collective life. In the fifth essay in Part II, I describe and make a critique of the main features of that ideology. There I postulate that it is not industrialism but the assumedly transcended category of capitalism that is the primary determinant of the nature of our society and of its system of medicine. In that respect, I question whether the inherent limitations and even iatrogeneses of medicine are primarily the result of its industrialization. Rather, I postulate that those limitations of medicine are given by its position within the class relations in contemporary capitalism. Its lack of effectiveness and iatrogeneses are determined by the very same forces that are responsible for the composition and functions of the health sector, i.e. the forces that determine contemporary capitalism, outlined in that essay and further detailed in Part III. Indeed, unless the dialectical relation between medicine and capitalism is understood, we cannot understand the limitations of and iatrogeneses of and in medicine.

The sixth essay in Part III provides an alternative explanation of the present composition, nature, and functions of the health sector in the United States to those frequently given in sociological, economic, and medical care literature. These explanations usually maintain that the American health sector is a result of the value system of the assumedly middle class American society. In this essay, it is postulated that the present economic structure of the United States determines and maintains a social class structure, both outside and within the health sector, and that the different degrees of ownership, control, and influence that these classes have on the means of production, reproduction, and legitimization in the United States explain the composition, nature, and functions of the health sector. It is further postulated that the value system is not the cause, but a symptom, of these class controls and influences. Also, those patterns of control and dominance are of paramount importance in understanding the feminization of the health labor force, the subject of the seventh essay in that part. Indeed, in order to comprehend why the majority of producers of medical services are women, we have to understand the situation of women within contemporary capitalism.

But, as Marx indicated, the point of the story is not only to explain reality, but to change it. How do we do this? This is an important question, and one whose urgency becomes all the more pressing with the realization that our Western system of power is in a state of profound crisis. To begin with, an understanding of political power and the nature of the state is of key importance. This is the subject of the lengthy eighth essay (Part IV), which is divided into three sections. Section I presents a critique of the contemporary theories of power, discussing the well-established countervailing pluralist and power elite theories, as well as those of bureaucratic and professional control, and also including a critique of those Marxist theories that have most frequently been debated in present times, i.e. economic determinism, structural determinism, and corporate statism. Section II discusses the role, nature, characteristics, and mode of intervention of the state, considered to be much in the center of the understanding of our reality. This section builds upon current debate, much enriched by the contributions of Gramsci, Miliband, Offe, Gough, O'Connor, Poulantzas, Althusser and others, to whom I am indebted.

Section III discusses the modus operandi of the state, a component of the analysis of political power and the nature of the state that has been greatly underdeveloped. There I present an expansion of that analysis, with specific focus on the mode of state intervention in contemporary developed capitalist societies, taking medicine as the arena of exposition. Also, I try in this section to explain the dramatic growth of the state intervention in the health sector, with an added analysis of the dialectical relationship between that growth and the fiscal crisis of the state. Both are intrinsically and dialectically related. In all three sections of this article, I have focused on Western European countries and on North America, choosing many of my examples and categories from the area of medicine.

Of course, the essays in this volume are not intended to provide a comprehensive critique of prevalent ideologies in the social sciences of medicine, or the detailed presentation of alternative ones. Rather, I consider them to be diagrams and sketches for alternative explanations to the asphyxiating patterns of orthodoxy prevalent today. In summary, I have aimed at showing that if we are to understand the ideology, nature, composition, distribution, and functions of the medical care sector in Western capitalist societies, we must first understand the forces that determine those societies. For that, I postulate that the assumedly transcended and diluted paradigms of capitalism, imperialism, social class and class struggle are far from being outmoded concepts of interest only to ideologues. Rather, they are categories of analysis much needed for our understanding of Western societies and their systems of medicine. They are, in summary, and as Neruda would put it, "at the center of things."

Needless to say, the interpretation of reality presented in this volume is a minority voice in our Western academic setting. It is in conflict with the prevalent explanations of the health sector, and this accounts for its exclusion from the realm of debate. Still, its veracity will be affirmed not by its "popularity" in the corridors of power, which will be nil, but in its verification on the terrain of practice and history.

Note on Tone and Style

In these essays, I have deliberately attempted to follow a discursive style, avoiding the baroque language that is so prevalent in academic circles on both sides of the ideological fence. Moreover, I have tried to rely heavily on empirical data to make theory more understandable and alive. The renaissance of Marxist studies in the Western world, liberated from the Stalinist shell, has been marked by a regrettable disregard for empirical research. The sterility of much bourgeois empiricism has led many radicals to indiscriminately castigate all factual inquiry as mindless empiricism. And, in that situation, the well-placed distaste for positivism and functionalism wrongly leads to a disregard for factual data. Fortunately, studies are now appearing that are breaking with such scholasticism and are making Marxism a widely comprehensible and accessible tool. I very much hope that this work further contributes to that end.

Acknowledgments

Having outlined the rationale for this volume, the themes covered and the style and tone used, it is only appropriate for me to end this introduction by acknowledging the assistance of many in shaping the positions presented in these pages. Indeed, whether wittingly or unwittingly, many have contributed to and influenced these essays. Presented on different occasions during the last five years, they owe much to discussions with friends and foes alike who helped shape their final form. Although written in the United States, they are based on past and present experiences in a number of other countries as well. In that respect, a list of acknowledgments may almost read as part of a biographical note.

First, thanks are due to my friends and compañeros of Catalonia and other nations of Spain, whose struggles against fascism I have shared since the 50s. They know and understand, better than most, my practical and theoretical origins. Their struggle, soon to be won, has been a splendid one. And their influence in stimulating and defining my life and work has been strong.

Also, many thanks are due to my friends in Italy, France, Sweden and Great Britain. The days, weeks, months and years that I lived with them are unforgettable. It was during that period in the early and middle 60s that I combined my practice in social medicine with my studies in social administration, political theory and political economy. Some among my European friends felt that I was wise in my interest in comprehensiveness. Others felt I was wrong. It may be for the reader of this volume to decide which group was right after all.

Thanks are also due to my friends of the Americas—North, Central and South. Since 1965, when I first arrived in the United States, I have had the opportunity to study, teach, work, struggle in and enjoy many parts, centers and institutions on both sides of the Rio Grande. And here is where I also owe to many—too many to be listed—my understanding and perceptions of the realities presented in these essays. From the southern part, I learned much from those who are today persecuted because of their belief that the only way of solving the underdevelopment of health is by breaking with the sickness of underdevelopment. They understand, better than most, the political nature of both health and medicine. From the northern part, I also learned from many. Here, a further personal note may be required. When I first came to the United States, I tried, somewhat formally, to learn the past and present of this beautiful country. But there, the dramatic insufficiency or the bluntly apologistic character of prevalent explanations of the U. S. reality and its power relations became quite apparent to me. There was a need to look for alternatives. And in the process of looking for alternatives, I found that there is much to learn from the unknown folk, from that history that is so well reflected in the poetry, songs and oral history of those who earn their living from their toil. It is plain to me that their story—the history of the working class of the U.S.—has not yet been written. But when it is, it will become quite clear that the history of the U.S. is a long, heartbreaking and impressive history of conflict and struggle. For helping me to understand it and be a participant in it, I owe much to many, and especially to the members of the study group on Capitalism and the seminar on Political Economy here at Hopkins. Thanks are particularly due to David Harvey for his stimulating friendship. I also wish to thank Grace Ziem, Elizabeth Fee, Hila Sherer, Sander Kelman, Len Rodberg, Robb Burlage, Howard Berliner, Knut Ringen, Janet Bouton, and many others of the East Coast Health Exchange Group for lively and productive discussions.

Last but not least, I benefited much from my own students. I learned much from them, from those with whom I had disagreements as much as agreements.

Finally, the production of a book is not possible without the work of many, whose contributions should not remain unrecognized. In that respect, I owe thanks to Debby Sarsgard, Janet Archer, and Christopher George for editing my English (with Catalan accent) manuscripts, to Jane Seitz for translating my unintelligible handwriting into a readable form, and to many other known and unknown persons who, by working in the production and distribution of this volume, have made it possible for my initial handwritten notes to appear in front of the reader.

The Johns Hopkins University, August, 1976.

PART I:
THE UNDERDEVELOPMENT OF
HEALTH IN CAPITALIST SOCIETIES

The Political and Economic Origins
of the Underdevelopment of
Health in Latin America

Oh love, oh my love,
tell me
are we poor because we do not have riches
or
is it that we don't have riches because we are poor?
(translated from an old Colombian folk song)

Assuming that a first step in analyzing the present maldistribution of human resources in the health sector of a country and a continent is to understand the nature of that condition and the reasons for it, I will focus in this paper on the causes of that maldistribution in our Americas, placing special emphasis on that part south of the Rio Grande—the Latin American continent—usually referred to as the underdeveloped America.[1] I am aware, of course, of the great diversity among the Latin American economies. However, I believe that all the Latin American countries (with the exception of Cuba) exhibit certain patterns of economic, social, and political structures and behaviors that, in the context of the distribution of resources, are more similar than dissimilar. I feel that these similarities justify the consideration of these different countries as a group in this paper.

Also, because the underdevelopment of poor nations is closely related to the development of the rich ones, I will also touch, although very briefly, upon the present maldistribution of human resources in the health sector of North America.

In addition, because, and as I will show, the distribution of human health resources follows and parallels the distribution of most of the resources in underdeveloped countries, I will analyze the distribution of resources in the health sector within the context of the parameters that determine underdevelopment and explain that distribution. In other words, I will examine the tree, the distribution of human health resources,

[1]The term "underdeveloped countries" will be used interchangeably in this paper with such terms as poor countries or nations and developing countries. At the same time, I am aware of the lack of a precise term that would define not only the state of poverty of the majority of our human race, but also the process that determines it. For an interesting discussion on this very point, see reference 1.

in the context of the forest, underdevelopment. Indeed, the thesis I will develop in this paper is that the present maldistribution of human health resources is brought about by the same determinants that cause the underdevelopment of Latin America.[2]

In so doing, I will try to close a gap in the ever increasing bibliography on health and health services in developing countries, which is rich in description but scarce in analysis. Indeed, in looking back on this large body of literature, we can see quite a number of scholarly and very elegant descriptive studies and reference works on the health and health services of developing countries. Yet, what most of these publications lack, as Ruderman (2) pointed out when he reviewed one of them, is an analytic explanation of why underdevelopment of health and health services came about in the first place. I would postulate that this omission is not an accidental one. Indeed, had they analyzed and begun to explain the underdevelopment of health and health services, those scholars and researchers might have come to the conclusion, uncomfortable as it may be, that the main cause of the underdevelopment of health was the state of health or lack of it, of the political, social, and economic structures that determine the underdevelopment in the societies studied. Avoidance of this analysis led these scholars to consider the maldistribution of health resources in a vacuum, as if this could be explained separately and independently from the analysis—admittedly sometimes embarrassing, and always sensitive—of those structures which determine that distribution to begin with.

Let me give an example. In the 1960s, a very thorough, elegant, and complete study—one of the most complete surveys that has ever been conducted, either in developed or developing countries—was carried out on the production and distribution of human health resources in Colombia (3). One finding of this study was that by social classes and by regions, the distribution of human health resources in that country was highly askew. Another fact brought out by this and other surveys was the highly skewed distribution of wealth and income in Colombia, with 5 per cent of the population owning 52 per cent of the wealth (4). It would have seemed logical to explore the possible correlation, and even causality, that might exist between the highly skewed distribution of wealth, income, and political power in that society and the highly skewed distribution of

[2]In my analysis of economic underdevelopment, I owe a great intellectual debt to André Gunder Frank, Paul Baran, and Charles Bettelheim. Actually, an intention of this paper is to show that their interpretative model of economic underdevelopment is also useful in explaining social underdevelopment in general and health resources underdevelopment in particular.

human health resources in the country. Yet, in a seminar arranged to discuss the meaning and conclusions of that health manpower study, and attended by prestigious scholars and researchers, not only was there no attempt to relate the distribution of wealth and human health resources, but the highly skewed distribution of wealth was not even mentioned, let alone discussed by these scholars (3). Oblivious and inattentive to the parameters within which this maldistribution of human health resources took place, their conclusions were empirically invalid and ineffective policy-wise.

The attitude detectable in this seminar reflects what Birnbaum (5) has called recently the tranquilizing effect of social research (and I would include a large percentage of health services research) in the 1960s. Indeed, social research in this period was characterized by the dominance of the empiricist, i.e. the expert on the trees who fails to see the forest.[3] It was the time, you may remember, when Daniel Bell wrote his *End of Ideology* (7), an end which, as Blackburn (8) indicates, was not so much the end but the victory of the ideology of empiricism and pragmatism.

This empiricism led the major part of studies on health services development and planning to emphasize the method, the method as the "unideologic," "value-free" instrument for distributing resources. Thus, the emphasis within the analysis, study, and application of the planning of the distribution of human health resources was on the methodologic aspects, without analyzing and/or questioning (but rather taking as "given") the social, economic, and political structures that determined and conditioned that underdevelopment. Cost-benefit, cost-effectiveness, PPBS, and the all-encompassing health planning CENDES method, were actually products of the "apologist" ideology that sustained those structures responsible for the maldistribution of resources.[4] A significant exception to this situation in Latin America was Cuba, which was exploring an alternative road to the one prevalent in Latin America for breaking with underdevelopment.

As for the rationale and explanation for underdevelopment, it was considered that the condition of Latin America was determined by the scarcity of resources. In this respect, the main assumption underlying the analysis of development has been that development is the transformation of one mode or type—the underdeveloped—to the other—the developed. In the analysis of development, the general features of the developed

---

[3] For a critique of empiricism and pragmatism, see reference 6.

[4] For a critique of the CENDES method and its limited application in Latin America, see reference 9.

countries are abstracted as an ideal type and compared or contrasted with the equally typical features of the poor societies. Development comes about, in this view, by the replacement of the features of the latter with those of the former. As a consequence of this interpretation, the model the underdeveloped countries are expected to follow contains all the features of the developed ones. Parsons (10), Hoselitz (11), and others have elaborated this model,[5] and recently Kahn and Weiner (13) have popularized it. Due to the great influence—and even control of ideas— that these sociologists and popularizers have enjoyed, their analyses have affected most writings on health services in underdeveloped countries. For instance, in a large number of references, most of the indicators of health services in underdeveloped countries, such as bed-population ratios, are compared with indicators from the developed ones, often accepting the premise that indicators of developed countries can be used as models or targets for the underdeveloped ones.[6]

A further elaboration of this approach can be seen in the "stages of growth" theory, popularized by Rostow's *Stages of Economic Growth* (16). According to Rostow, development is the process whereby a country changes its characteristics in five stages. The writer assumes the stages to be universal and to apply to all countries.

Because of the great influence that the Rostowian interpretation of development has enjoyed, it merits examination in some detail.

It is possible to identify all societies, in their economic dimensions, as lying within five categories: the traditional society, the preconditions for take-off, the take-off, the drive to maturity, and the age of high mass-consumption. First, the traditional society. A traditional society is one whose structure is developed within limited production functions, based on pre-Newtonian science and technology, and on pre-Newtonian attitudes towards the physical world. . . . The second stage of growth embraces societies in the process of transition; that is, the period when the preconditions for take-off are developed; for it takes time to transform a traditional society in the ways necessary for it to exploit the fruits of modern science to fend off diminishing returns, and thus to enjoy the blessings and choices opened up by the march of compound interest. . . . the stage of preconditions arise(s) not endogenously but from some external intrusion by more advanced societies. . . . We come now to the great watershed in the life of modern societies: the third stage in this sequence, the take-off. The take-off is the interval when the old blocks and resistances to steady growth are finally overcome. The forces

[5] For a thorough and critical review of the U.S. sociology of development, see reference 12.
[6] For a representative study using this analysis, see reference 14. For an excellent critique of this approach, see reference 15.

making for economic progress, which yielded limited bursts and enclaves of modern activity, expand and come to dominate the society. Growth becomes its normal condition. Compound interest becomes built, as it were, into its habits and institutional structure. . . . [The] take-off is defined as requiring all three of the following related conditions: (1) a rise in the rate of productive investment from, say, 5 percent or less to over 10 percent of national income (or net national product (NNP)); (2) the development of one or more substantial manufacturing sectors, with a high rate of growth; (3) the existence or quick emergence of a political, social and institutional framework which exploits the impulses to expansion . . . (17).

In the Rostow interpretative model, the major factor in development is contained in his third or take-off stage, and this is characterized by a rapid rate of investment and growth.

Rostow visualizes two major agents of change, determinants of the process of development. The first agent of change identified is the *diffusion of values* (entrepreneurial values) from the developed societies or metropolises to the underdeveloped societies, initially to the national capitals of the underdeveloped societies, then to their provincial capitals, and finally to the peripheral hinterlands. Development is thus perceived as a phenomenon of acculturation and diffusion of institutional and organizational values, together with the transmission of skills, knowledge, and technology, from the developed to the developing countries.

The second agent of change is the *diffusion of capital.* According to Rostow and the previously mentioned authors, the underdeveloped countries are poor because they lack investment capital and therefore cannot develop and escape from their poverty. As a consequence of this assumption, they believe it essential for the development of the poor countries that the richer, developed countries diffuse capital to the underdeveloped ones, thereby stimulating their economic development. Thus, foreign capital, according to the Rostowian interpretation, creates a "market, entrepreneurial economy" in the form of an "enclave," similar to the one in the developed or metropolis society, which evolves first in the poor nation's capital, and from there expands its positive and economically stimulating influence to the rest of the country.

This interpretation leads the authors to the conclusion that development takes place in, is stimulated by, and is channeled through an "enclave" of the developed, metropolitan economy within each of the underdeveloped countries. Indeed, they consider that there are dual economies in the underdeveloped countries: one, the "enclave," urban-based, well developed market economy, with technical, entrepreneurial, and cultural values diffused from the developed metropolis; and the other, "the marginal economy" that includes those rural-based sectors of the population, sometimes its majority, that have not been incorporated into the "entrepreneurial market economy."

Because of the great influence of the Rostowian school of thought in the sociology of underdevelopment, inside as well as outside the health sector, the three characteristics of the Rostowian theory, i.e. (a) the need for cultural and technologic diffusion, (b) the scarcity of national capital, and (c) the dual economies, all appear in most of the literature dealing with distribution of general resources, and also human health resources, in developing countries.[7]

Indeed, the *cultural diffusion* argument is reflected, in health services literature, in the heavy emphasis placed on the necessity of training different types of personnel in underdeveloped countries following the curriculum and educational resources prevalent in the developed countries. The second Rostowian argument, on the *scarcity of capital,* is presented with different interpretations but usually appears under the rubric "that poor countries *cannot afford* to provide whole health care to the whole population" or also under the argument that poor countries can "only afford social security for a few sectors, and mainly the industrial urban based sector, because investment capital determines the overall important growth of the take-off stage." The concept of *dual economies and societies* is reflected in the existence of an unequal distribution of health resources between the cities and the rural hinterlands, with Western "hospital-based" medicine in the cities and the indigenous and "less developed" form of medicine in the rural areas. This dualism is considered to have come about, first, because of the lack of diffusion of Western developed medicine to the rural areas (argument 1 of the Rostowian interpretation) and, second, because of the lack of resources and investment capital in those areas (argument 2).

Rostow's "stages of growth" theory is the most accepted theory for explaining development and analyzing the distribution of resources, both within and outside the health sector. Its popularity in the corridors of power and academic circles in developed countries (as well as in the leading circles in developing countries and in the international agencies) is attributable partially to its rationalization and justification of the present relationship between the developed and the developing nations, present-ing the developed countries as "models" to be emulated by poor countries and showing underdevelopment to be due to an assumed

[7]For the most comprehensive, empirical study of the "stages theory" of social (including health services) and economic development, see reference 14.

scarcity of resources in underdeveloped areas and not to economic structures and the pattern of economic relationships between poor and rich countries. The "fault" of underdevelopment is therefore left squarely on the shoulders of the poorer nations.

The Fallacy of Some of the Theories of Underdevelopment Currently Popular Inside and Outside the Health Sector

Frank (18), Baran (19), and Griffin (20), however, have all shown the Rostowian model and its derivatives to be empirically invalid when confronted with reality, and to be theoretically inadequate when called upon to explain the process of development and its concurrent distribution of resources. This inadequacy explains why such theories are ineffective policy-wise for promoting development.

Let us analyze each of the three basic postulates of the Rostowian theory and check them against the empirical evidence available to us from sources outside the health sector, as well as from data gathered within the health services.

First, regarding the supposed lack of diffusion of cultural values, available evidence shows that, quite contrary to the Rostowian assumption, there is a very large diffusion—so much so that some may even refer to it as dominance—of cultural values abstracted from or generated from developed to developing societies. As several authors have pointed out, the media (television and the press) in Latin America are on the whole very heavily influenced by the values of North America. As Frank (21) notes, in Mexico the Spanish version of the *Reader's Digest*, for instance, has a higher circulation than the entire circulations of Mexico's eight largest magazines put together. And, according to a recent UNESCO report (22), 70 per cent of the TV programs shown in Latin America originate in the United States.

Another important element of cultural diffusion is institutional education. The system of primary, secondary, and university education, patterned after the systems in developed countries, is usually alien to the needs of poor countries. A recent UNESCO report (23) states, for instance, that while most inhabitants of underdeveloped nations live in agricultural, rural sectors where there is a need for a collective sense of solidarity, most of the values expounded in primary and secondary schools are urban, and are, as in most Western developed societies, individually, entrepreneurially, and urban-oriented. Cultural diffusion also takes place at the university level. As Garcia (24) has shown, in a comprehensive review of medical education in Latin America, most medical curricula in Latin America have been patterned on German, French, Spanish, and, more recently, American models, and these are models that, as McKeown (25) has indicated, reflect an engineering approach to the understanding of the body and its diseases and tend to ignore the understanding of the socioeconomic environment that brought about the diseases. The emphasis on hospital-based, technologically-oriented medicine and especially individual, acute-episodic care, typical of the medical education of Western developed societies, is replicated in the developing societies. Rural, ambulatory, social, and continuous care is underrepresented, if not nonexistent, in the curricula of medical institutions in developing societies. When the rural type of medical care is taught, student exposure is apt to be more symbolic than real (26).

Thus, quite contrary to the Rostowian claim, there is a very heavy diffusion of cultural values from developed to developing countries. Moreover, it can be postulated, again contrary to Rostow's assumption, that this cultural diffusion—defined by Candau, the late Director-General of the World Health Organization, as "cultural imperialism"—is, as I will try to show later on, more harmful than beneficial to the process of development.

Complementing this observable cultural diffusion is technologic diffusion. Let me underline, incidentally, that I believe false the dichotomy commonly drawn between cultural diffusion and technologic diffusion. Indeed, technology is a value-laden (and not value-free) process in which cultural values are assumed and subsumed. According to the United Nations Economic Committee for Latin America (UN-ECLA), most of the technology of Latin America has been imported from the developed areas, and primarily from North America. Actually, Fucaraccio (27) has stated that 80 per cent of Latin American equipment is imported. And, as Illich (28) has indicated, this technology, which is foreign to the parameters of underdevelopment, can harm more than benefit the process of development. The labor-saving technology of developed society actually contributes to the creation of unemployment in the underdeveloped countries.[8] Moreover, the investment needed for this technology diverts vital investment from less glamorous, but more efficient and much more needed projects. Not long ago I estimated, for example, that with the annual operating expenditures of the three open-

[8]For an analysis of the harmful effects of Western technology on the economies of Latin America, see reference 29.

heart surgery units in use today in Bogotá, a city with a population of over 2 million, a quarter of the children living there could receive a half-liter of milk each day for one year. I should underline here that the main public health problems in the city of Bogotá are not heart conditions but gastroenteritis, infectious diseases, and malnutrition (30). Furthermore, if indeed the experience of developed countries applies to developing ones, it is highly probable that, considering the high density of units for such a small catchment area, the care provided by these units is not really needed.

Once again, to refute Rostow's theory, it can be postulated that there is too much, rather than too little, cultural and technologic diffusion from the developed to the developing countries.

The Myth of the Scarcity of Resources

As for the second Rostowian assumption, on the lack of capital and the need for more capital investment by developed nations in the developing countries, several authors have shown that the Rostowian model is inaccurate as an explicative model of underdevelopment. Indeed, Fucaraccio (27), and others (31), have shown that there is no scarcity of capital in Latin America, but rather an underuse and misuse of capital. Fucaraccio points out that Colombia and Argentina, for instance, invest 20 per cent and 23 per cent of their domestic gross national products, respectively, which compares quite favorably to the lower percentages of 16 per cent and 18 per cent invested by the U.S. and France in their respective domestic economies. But, for an analysis of the ramifications of a country's investment process, the nature and control of investment is more important than the size of investment.

As for the nature of these investments, a large proportion is financed from domestic savings. This leads to the question of which people are saving. To answer this question, it is necessary to examine the levels of income distribution in Latin America, where

> . . . (a) a large part of income is concentrated in a minority of the population . . . which generates the savings subsequently converted into capital goods; and (b) at least 50 percent of the population not only do not have the ability to save but lack sufficient income even to satisfy their most basic needs which are estimated at about $190 per annum per capita (27).

This distribution of income and corresponding use of savings determines the structure of investments, production, and consumption, where

. . . the construction sector accounts for between 40 and 50 per cent of gross domestic investment, depending on the year and the country concerned. A considerable part of such construction represents residential units which do little to solve the low-income housing shortage in Latin America and in no way help to increase productive capacity. The remainder comprises construction related to productive capacity and to public works. Equipment accounts for between 50 and 60 per cent of investment, of which half is for transportation and the remainder machinery and spare parts.

This distribution of investment suggests that Latin America could increase its rate of growth and assume a less vulnerable position if it were to change its pattern of investment accordingly. However, since the pattern of investment is conditioned by the pattern of savings, which in turn is conditioned by income distribution, a substantial modification in the pattern of investment could mean breaking the rules under which the system operates, insofar as it may conflict with the criteria of profitability.

Also, there is a quite marked underutilization of capital, the factor allegedly in scarce supply. According to an ILPES-CELADE (UN-Latin American Institute for Socio-Economic Planning-Latin American Commission for Development) study, between 1960 and 1963, only 58.2 percent of industrial productive capacity was utilized. This situation, which tends to perpetuate itself, is attributed to distribution and levels of income and to causes of a technologic nature (27).

Furthermore, the emergence of the highly controlled economy in the international economic sphere has resulted in strong links between domestic and foreign capital, and this has constituted a relationship that has meant an external decapitalization, where private investment, as the Foreign Ministers of Latin America (except Cuba) indicated in the Viña del Mar meeting in 1969 (32), has meant,

. . . and now means, that the sums taken out of our [Latin American] countries are several times higher than the amounts invested. Our potential capital is being reduced. The profits on investment grow and multiply, not in our countries but abroad. So-called aid, with all the well-known restrictions attached to it, means markets and further development for the developed countries, but it does not compensate for the sums which leave Latin America as payment for external indebtedness or as profits produced by direct private investment. In a word, we know that Latin America gives more than it receives.

Contrary to Rostow's thesis, the diffusion of capital does not go from developed to developing countries, but rather, from developing to developed. In 1969, the same year the Foreign Ministries meeting took place, U.S. companies took out of Latin America roughly $1 billion more in profits than they invested there (33). And as Frank (21, p. 50) has noted, the largest part of the capital

> . . . which the developed countries own in the underdeveloped ones was never sent from the former to the latter at all but was, on the contrary acquired by the developed countries in the now underdeveloped ones.

The Flow of Human Capital in the Health Sector from Developing to Developed Countries

Here, again, reflecting what occurs in other sectors of the economy, there is a pattern of diffusion and flow of human health resources from Latin America to North America that represents a savings for the North American economy. Indeed, it has been estimated that the overall saving for the U.S. as a result of the inflow of 5756 physicians from developing countries in 1971 was equivalent to the yearly output from fully half of the 120 U.S. medical schools (34).

Foreign-trained doctors presently represent 20 per cent of all practicing physicians in the United States, and some states have a higher proportion, e.g. New York, with 38 per cent (35). In some specialties and types of practice these percentages are higher still. For instance, preliminary data from a recent survey of mental hospitals conducted by the American Psychiatric Association, indicated that two-thirds of filled psychiatric positions were held by foreign-trained physicians (35). All before-mentioned figures, incidentally, include only permanent U.S. residents and exclude interns, residents, fellows, and exchange visitors. When we include all these categories, then, the annual inflow of foreign physicians who entered the United States in 1970, 1971, and 1972 was far greater than the number the country produced in each one of those years (36). Of those who stayed and became permanent residents during the decade 1960-1970, 35 per cent came from Latin America (37), representing an annual direct and indirect savings during that period of approximately $400 million—a superior amount to the annual "aid" in medical care and hospitals that went from the U.S. to Latin America in the same time period, estimated to be $20 million (38). It is worth underlining that this medical "aid" is mainly focused on teaching hospitals, perpetuating the pattern of production that benefits the consumption of the donor country and of those groups in the recipient country that Frank calls the lumpenbourgeoisie. (By lumpenbourgeoisie is meant those domestic social groups in underdeveloped societies that control most of the wealth of their society and who, at the same time, have identical interests to those of foreign industry and commerce. The expression "lumpen" is added to the term bourgeoisie because their economic, social, and political power is dependent on the power of the bourgeoisie of the metropolis (18, p. 5).

The pattern of production prevalent in the health sector of developing countries, as we will see later, is hospital-based, technologic and specialized medicine relevant to the needs of the lumpenbourgeoisie but not to the majority of the population.

The exodus of human health resources implies a very serious decapitalization for each donor country. Ozlak and Caputo (36) have estimated that the annual loss for the whole of Latin America due to the flow of physicians to the United States is $200 million, a figure which is equal to Chile's education budget for 1970, or to the total medical aid given by the United States to Latin America throughout the decade of the 1960s. This decapitalization is particularly accentuated in some countries, such as the Dominican Republic, where one-half of that nation's newborn children die before reaching the age of five, and from which country 30 per cent of medical school graduates each year emigrate to the United States (39).

The Causes of Underdevelopment of Human Resources Inside and Outside the Health Sector

The main reason for underdevelopment in Latin America, as a recent UN-ECLA report (40) states, is the nature, subject, and control of economic and social investment leading to a pattern of production and consumption aimed at optimizing the benefits of the foreign and national controllers of that capital, and not at stimulating the equitable distribution of resources in the particular Latin American nations. The report emphasizes that these patterns of investment

> . . . determine a structure of production in the modern sector which is mainly characterized by the production of consumer goods, particularly consumer durables of a luxury type. Even the relatively small scale production of capital goods is designed to reinforce production machinery that is geared to consumption, to the detriment of a possible expansion of the capital goods sector which might boost the development of the rest of the economy and ensure its ultimate capacity for self-sustained development.

Also, in another UN-ECLA report (41) it is said that

. . . the establishment or expansion of a sector of consumer durables or luxury goods, such as automobiles, television sets, or refrigerators—the base of mass consumption in developed countries—tends to depend upon the expansion and broadening of credit and loan facilities. In substance, savings and cash assets of various types, including foreign loans, are absorbed by these activities and diverted from a hypothetical, direct role in the formation of productive capital.

These patterns of production and consumption repeat themselves throughout the primary, secondary, and tertiary sectors of the economy, with the tertiary sector, including health services and education, supporting the secondary and primary sectors. Furthermore, within the tertiary sector (as with the other two sectors), the public sector is, on the whole, aimed at strengthening the private sector.

Indeed, parallel to what occurs in the overall economy, the same social groups that determine the patterns of production and consumption in the primary and secondary sectors also shape patterns of production and consumption in the health sector. And it can be posited that these are patterns that do not benefit the majority of the population. In addition, as in other economic sectors, the public sector exists to take care of and strengthen (some may say so as to avoid its collapse) the private sector. Finally, the overall cause of the lack of health services coverage of the whole population is not the scarcity of capital and resources in the health sector, but the maldistribution and misuse of those resources.

The Fallacy of Underdevelopment

In summary, the cause of underdevelopment and its consequent maldistribution of resources is not (a) the scarcity of the proper "values" and technology in poor countries, (b) the scarcity of capital, and (c) the insufficient diffusion of capital, values and technology from developed society to the underdeveloped country's enclave and from the enclave to the rural areas, but quite the opposite. The cause of underdevelopment in poor nations is precisely the existence of Rostow's "conditions for development" in these countries. That is, (a) too much cultural and technologic dependency, and (b) the underuse and poor use of existing capital by certain national and international groups who have control of those resources. Moreover, factors (a) and (b) determine factor (c), the "dual economies" with the advanced, urban-based entrepreneurial market sector and the underdeveloped, rural-based, "non-market" marginal sector. The so-called "marginal" and "market" sectors of the economy, in fact, are intrinsically linked, so one cannot explain one sector without explicating the other. The development of the "market" model is determined by the underdevelopment of the "marginal" form. Indeed, the wealth of the enclave is based on the surplus generated by the "marginal" rural sector. And contrary to Rostow's assumption, it is the intrusion of the values of the developed countries, along with their technology and "entrepreneurial, market, international" capital into the poor societies, that creates the source of underdevelopment. As Frank (21, p. 8) has shown, the regions that are most underdeveloped and that seem today the most feudal

> . . . are the ones which had the closest ties to the metropolis in the past. They are the regions which were the greatest exporters of primary products and the biggest sources of capital for the world metropolis and were abandoned by the metropolis when for one reason or another business fell off. This hypothesis also contradicts the generally held thesis that the source of a region's underdevelopment is its isolation and its pre-capitalist institutions.

Frank further explains that this is illustrated by

> . . . the former super-satellite development and present ultra-under-development of the once sugar-exporting West Indies, Northeastern Brazil, the ex-mining districts of Minas Gerais in Brazil, highland Peru, and Bolivia, and the central Mexican states of Guanajuato, Zacatecas, and others whose names were made world famous centuries ago by their silver. There surely are no major regions in Latin America which are today more cursed by underdevelopment and poverty; yet all of these regions, like Bengal in India, once provided the life blood of mercantile and industrial capitalist development in the metropolis. These regions' participation in the development of the world capitalist system gave them, already in their golden age, the typical structure of underdevelopment of a capitalist export economy. When the market for their sugar or the wealth of their mines disappeared and the metropolis abandoned them to their own devices, the already existing economic, political, and social structure of these regions prohibited autonomous generation of economic development and left them no alternative but to turn in upon themselves and to degenerate into the ultra-underdevelopment we find there today.

Despite the claims of the Rostowian theories of underdevelopment popular in the United States, the main cause of underdevelopment is control of the economy by a small percentage of the population, Frank's lumpenbourgeoisie, which has strong connections with international capital and close affinity to the values, tastes and forms of consumption typical in the developed countries. It is this group which establishes and determines the pattern of production and consumption in underdeveloped societies, and which molds a pattern of production and consumption that is not conducive to, nor is it aimed at, the overall development of those societies.

An example of the power of the lumpenbourgeoisie can be seen in the automobile industry. Prebisch (42) has commented:

> What happened in the automobile industry was instructive. Not only did several countries attempt to do the same thing, but there was also an extraordinary proliferation of uneconomic plants in one country. In addition to Argentina and Brazil, countries which at present have real production, there are four other countries—Colombia, Mexico, Chile, and Venezuela—which maintain assembly plants and are preparing to begin production. The total Latin American market for passenger vehicles—estimated at little more than 300,000 units annually—has to be divided among nearly 40 present and potential manufacturers, while each of the principal European manufacturers delivers 250,000 to 500,000 units to the market annually.

It has been estimated that the annual value of automobile production in Argentina in the middle-1960s could in five years double the country's road network and

> . . . that a much more complete system of public transportation could be provided if only a part of this same amount were invested in buses and trucks instead of in private cars for the affluent minority (43).

Also, that

> . . . costs of both "foreign" and national investment in an industry like the automobile industry lead to greater underdevelopment. They result in underutilization of national resources, improper use of resources which might have been more adequately employed in promoting self-sustaining economic development, deepening inequalities in the distribution of national income, and the creation by these industries of vested economic, social, and political interests which are committed to continuing policies of underdevelopment. All this has an unfavorable effect on other existing industries and on the national economy as a whole (18, p. 111).

Thus the consumption patterns of the lumpenbourgeoisie and the middle class, stimulated by a "value system" aimed at producing a consumer society with Western, middle class standards of living (which would come about in the last stage of the Rostowian process of development), divert capital from potential investment. It should be added that in Latin America the lumpenbourgeoisie and middle class make up only between 15 and 20 per cent of the population (44), and the majority of the people, who are not of lumpenbourgeoisie and middle class level, do not fully participate in the consumer society. In a similar manner to that observed by Marcuse (45) in developed societies, the majority of the population is made to aspire to "more," where "more" is always unattainable.

Let me state here that I group the middle class with the lumpenbourgeoisie because, in agreement with an increasing number of social critics, I believe that economically the middle class functions as a dependent group to the lumpenbourgeoisie. In this respect, a UN-ECLA report (46) states that "the middle class in Latin America . . . improved their social status by coming to terms with the oligarchy." Indeed, throughout the underdeveloped countries, as Kolko (47) has also shown for the U.S., when the income of the middle class rises, it increases at the expense of the large masses of poor and near poor, not at the expense of the lumpenbourgeoisie (21, p. 39).

The pattern of consumption of the lumpenbourgeoisie and middle class, meant to benefit a limited percentage of the population, can also be seen in the distribution of health resources. Accordingly, the distribution of health resources follows an inverse relationship to the need for them. This maldistribution, by type of care, by region, by social class and by the type of financing, is determined by those same parameters that define the evident socioeconomic underdevelopment, which I examined in the preceding sections.

The Prevalent Patterns of Consumption: Imbalance by Type of Care

The use made by the population of Colombia of the available health services, according to the 1965-1966 health manpower survey previously mentioned (3), was such that for a period of two weeks, out of each group of 1,000 people, 387 of whom were defined as sick, 63 were under the care of an ambulatory physician and 2 under hospital care (24, p. 143). Comparing this distribution of need and utilization of health services, very likely similar in most Latin American countries, with the actual consumption of resources as measured by expenditures in several countries, shown in Table 1, we see that the pattern of public consumption of the Colombian health peso is such that the two hospital patients consume approximately 30 per cent of the health peso in the public sector and the 63 ambulatory patients about 60 per cent (with all

Table 1

Estimated health expenditures of the public health sector in medical care and water and sewerage supply per capita and by percentages of total health expenditures[ab]

| Country | Year | Medical Care[c] | | Water and Sewerage | | Total | |
		Per Capita Expenditures (U.S.$)[d]	Per cent[d]	Per Capita Expenditures (U.S.$)[d]	Per cent[d]	Per Capita Expenditures (U.S.$)[d]	Per cent[d]
Colombia	1970	8.5	91.2	0.82	8.8	9.32	100
Nicaragua	1969	14.6	94.4	0.86	5.6	15.46	100
Peru	1969	10.6	94.2	0.65	5.8	11.25	100
El Salvador	1970	6.1	94.4	0.36	5.6	6.46	100
Venezuela	1970	38.6	95.6	1.79	4.4	40.39	100

[a] Source, reference 48.

[b] If instead of considering only expenditures of the public sector on medical care, we consider estimations of total expenditures in medical care (public sector plus private sector), the percentages of expenditures in water and sewerage would be as follows: Colombia, 4.4–6 per cent; Peru, 1:5–4.7 per cent; El Salvador, 0.2–2.1 per cent; and Venezuela, 4–23 per cent.

[c] Data on distribution of expenditures in medical care between primary, secondary, and tertiary care are available only for Chile (Study of Human Resources. Chilean Ministry of Public Health, Santiago, 1970), and are partially available for Peru (Hall, T. Study of Human Resources. Johns Hopkins Press, Baltimore, 1971). Extracted from these sources are the following data on medical services expenditures: Chile (1968), ambulatory, 13.4 per cent; dental, 17.9 per cent; laboratory, 4.3 per cent; hospitalization, 9.4 per cent; and pharmaceutical, 55 per cent. In Peru (1964), 29 per cent of expenditures were for pharmaceutical costs.

[d] Source, Annual Report of the Director, 1971. Pan American Health Organization, Washington, D.C., 1971. From the total amount invested between January 1961–December 1970, an annual mean of investments has been obtained, and from this, per capita expenditures have been calculated.

types of curative services taking up around 91.2 per cent of the peso). In comparison, environmental services (including operating and capital expenditures), only consume 8 per cent of the Colombian health peso in that sector (48). When the private consumption is added to the public one, the percentage of overall consumption for environmental services is even lower, being between 4.4 per cent and 5 per cent. The situation is similar in other Latin American countries.

If we look at the type of morbidity prevalent in the surveyed population (i.e. infectious diseases and malnutrition) and at the comparative effectiveness of the different health activities for combating this morbidity, it would seem that environmental health services and preventive personal health services should be given far higher priority than curative services, and particularly the hospital services. In spite of this, the production of human resources, through the medical education imported from developed societies, serves to perpetuate this hospital-oriented, curative medicine approach which only strengthens the maldistribution of resources according to type of care by replicating the consumption of health resources prevalent in developed societies (49).

Imbalance in consumption by type of health care is also apparent in the distribution of health manpower according to specialties. Table 2 shows the percentage distribution of physicians, by specialty, for the United States and for three Latin American countries.

The distribution of specialties is very similar in both the developing and the developed countries represented here. Actually, in twelve Latin American countries, surgery represents the top specialty by percentage of physicians, with pediatrics and public health being the lowest categories. It should be obvious that there is an oversupply of the former specialty, and—in countries with 48 per cent of their population under 15 years of age and morbidity mainly caused by environmental and nutritional deficiencies—an undersupply of the latter specialties.

The orientation toward a hospital-based, curative medicine pattern of consumption seen in developed societies is replicated, through the medical education and the structure of health services, in underdeveloped countries, because the means of production and consumption in the health sector are controlled by the lumpenbourgeoisie, which desires the same type of care (with the "latest" in medical care) given to the people in developed lands. Due to the emigration of physicians from developing to

Table 2

Percentage distribution of physicians by some specialties[a]

Country	Year	General Practice	Public Health	Surgery	Pediatrics
Argentina	1969	8.9	—	26.7	8.6
Ecuador	1970	45.8	—	17.8	8.4
Paraguay	1971	8.2	0.7	15.2	8.0
United States	1970	17.8	0.8	20.0	6.0

[a] Source, *Health Manpower in the Americas*. Department of Human Resources, Pan American Health Organization, Washington, D.C., 1973.

developed societies described earlier, this pattern of production of human resources also benefits consumers in the metropolis.

It is also worth noting that the patterns of production and consumption in the metropolises or developed societies also are not aimed at meeting the needs of the majority of their population. As Bettelheim (50) indicates, the pattern of economic and social production and consumption of developing countries, and the consequent economic and social dependency, concerns only the bourgeoisie of both types of societies, and does not benefit the majority of the population in either. This can be clearly seen in the distribution of human health resources by type of health care. Indeed, Table 2 shows a distribution of resources unfavorable to the pattern of need in both societies. Also, it should be noted that the decapitalization of human resources in the underdeveloped country does not necessarily benefit the majority of the population in the developed nation. In fact, as Stevens and Vermeulen (37) have shown, most immigrant physicians in the United States tend to concentrate in already overserved areas and very few practice in the underserved areas of that country.

This pattern of consumption by type of care, in both developing and developed countries, is characterized by the broadening of choice for the few, and the narrowing of choice for the many. Actually, as the prestigious Chilean economist de Ahumada (51) has indicated, each dollar spent in Latin America on highly specialized hospital services costs a hundred lives. Had each dollar been spent on providing safe drinking water and in supplying food to the population, a hundred lives could have been saved. However hyperbolic Ahumada's statement may sound, it nevertheless provides a devastating critique of the pattern of investment in most developing countries.

Regional Imbalance

The important political and economic influence the city-based lumpen-bourgeoisie has on the distribution of resources also means that most of the human health resources are centered on the poor country's "enclave" of the market foreign-oriented economy. Thus, although most of the economic production is in the non-enclave areas, the agricultural and extraction sectors, the consumption of services, including human health resources, is urban and is primarily in the underdeveloped country's capital.

Table 3 compares the distribution of human health resources by

Table 3

Distribution of population and number of physicians per 10,000 inhabitants in some Latin American countries[a]

Country	Year[c]	Physicians Per 10,000	Localities Less Than 20,000 Population		Localities 20,000-99,999 Population		Localities More than 100,000 Population[b]	
			Physicians Per 10,000	Per cent of Population	Physicians Per 10,000	Per cent of Population	Physicians Per 10,000	Per cent of Population
Colombia	1970 (1964)	5.4	0.78	63.9	2.10	9.5	15.1	26.6
Nicaragua	1971 (1969)	4.5	1.37	72.6	11.2	8.6	13.8	18.8
Peru[d]	1969 (1961)	5.2	(1.6)	76.0	(1.6)	16.8	14.5	7.2
El Salvador	1969	2.3	2.64	81.1	6.2	5.1	11.1	13.3

[a] Source, reference 48. Data taken from *Quadrennial Projections*, 1971. Pan American Health Organization, Washington, D.C., 1971.
[b] Includes national capitals: Bogota (1967), 13.7 physicians per 10,000 people; Managua (1971), 13.8 physicians per 10,000 people. In 1969, El Salvador had only two cities over 100,000 inhabitants, the capital, San Salvador, being one of these.
[c] Figures in parentheses refer to the census years in which the listed population distributions were determined.
[d] Figures for physicians per 10,000 people in Peru are for localities with less than 100,000 inhabitants.

community size in different countries and shows that those resources are concentrated not in the small communities, where most of the people live, but in the large cities and primarily in the capital.

The lumpenbourgeoisie influences the distribution of resources by: (a) Stressing the "market model" in the distribution of resources, in the same way that it expounds a "liberal ideology" at the economic level. Resources are thus distributed according to consuming, not producing power.[9] This consumer power, as indicated before, is urban-based. (b) Influence on the means of production, i.e. urban-based medical education. As Freidson (53) has stated, "A profession attains and maintains its position by virtue of the protection and patronage of some elite segment of society which has been persuaded that there is some special value in its work." (c) Control of the social content and nature of the medical profession, due to the unavailability and inaccessibility to the majority of the population of university education (24, p. 200); and (d) control of the highly centralized, urban-based State organs, whereby the public sector, controlled by the different branches of the State,[10] is basically meant to support the private and social security sectors.

The Consequences of the Enclave Theory in the Health Sector

Private and social security sectors take care of considerable parts of the urban-based lumpenbourgeoisie and middle classes, with the public sector taking care of the majority of the population, either the lumpenproletariat in the urban areas or the peasantry in the rural areas, which together constitute 70 per cent of the Latin American population (44). This distribution of resources seems to reflect the dual-economy theory of Rostow. Indeed, you will recall, within the Rostowian theory, that the third or take-off stage was Rostow's stage for the change from a primitive or traditional society to a consumer-oriented society. This take-off takes place through investment (primarily in the industrial sector) in the underdeveloped countries. In this process of development the country moves toward the features of the developed countries, predicting for the developing countries a future similar to that of the wealthy ones. Within

[9] For an excellent analysis of the parameters that define the market model, see reference 52.

[10] The State includes the following institutions: the government, the administration, the military and police, the judicial branch, and the parliamentary assemblies, all of whose interrelationships determine the form of the state system (54).

this interpretation, the industrial sector is the dynamic factor in the Latin American economy. As Roemer (55) says,

> . . . the economic development of a country depends upon industrialization. Even the improvement of agriculture depends largely on the production of farm machinery, transport, fertilizer, and other items requiring industrial processes. Thus, it is reasonable for a developing country to give priority in health resource allocation to its industrial workers. A skilled industrial worker represents a social investment; that is, the attainment of the skill ordinarily requires long training and experience.

As a result of this human investment theory, the investment of resources should be based on the industrial sector. Roemer continues:

> Thus, it seems to me that in countries of all types—industrialized and developing, capitalist and socialist—the social insurance mechanism is virtually an inevitable stage in the political and economic process of attaining effective distribution of personal health services to a total population. In the course of this evolution there may well be temporary inequities, favoring certain social groups as compared with others, but this is in the very nature of social progress. It is realistically not a great price to pay for the advantages of stability, planning, the achievement of a higher priority for health, and all the other advantages of the social insurance approach discussed earlier.

This interpretation, however, does not correspond to the dynamics of the development currently observable in Latin America. Actually, as UN-ECLA (56) has shown, the industrial sector is not a dynamic factor in the Latin American economy.

> Industry has ceased to be a driving force in the Latin American economy; instead, it has simply become one of the number of sectors with no special power to galvanize the others.

As indicated before (and also as pointed out by UN-ECLA, Frank, and very many others), the pattern of investments in this sector is aimed at sustaining the consumer goods industry rather than establishing a force for economic development. The control of that investment by the lumpenbourgeoisie and its foreign counterparts optimizes the pattern of investments that diverts capital from actual development purposes. Also, and as Frank (18, p. 119) notes, the same productive processes and structures which promote underdevelopment also produce high incomes for the Latin American bourgeoisie. The industrial sector then is controlled by and functions for the lumpenbourgeoisie and its foreign counterparts, not for the benefit of the development of the whole of the individual country. Furthermore, even though this sector served as a stimulant for development in North America and Europe, it is not a dynamic sector in Latin America because, unlike those two continents, the Latin American continent lacks a great internal demand that can sustain its industrial sector. The difference between Latin America and those other areas is that in North American and in Europe industrialization did not precede, but followed, profound structural changes and reforms, primarily in agriculture, which determined an internal demand that sustained the process of industrialization. As Feder (57), a consultant to UN-ECLA and UN-FAO, has pointed out, the main obstacle to industrialization and development in Latin America is the system of land ownership, and the lack of meaningful land reform which could create such an internal demand.

Because of its lack of dynamism, the industrial sector has remained stagnant, and it employed the same percentage of the labor force (14 per cent) from 1950 to 1969. In addition, and reflecting this stagnation, social security coverage for the middle sectors—professionals, white and blue-collar workers—has remained rather constant in the last decade, and has exhibited very slow, if any, expansion. Table 4 shows the percentage of population covered by social security in various countries, in different time periods. Actually, all the increase in Latin American social security coverage has concerned the services sector (primarily the group comprising government employees), which has been the fastest growing sector in Latin America. In 1969, 43 per cent of the labor force was in services (18, p. 52).

It is therefore highly questionable whether, as long as the pattern of control in those sectors remains the same, the industrial (and services) sector can be the dynamic multiplier it has been assumed to be. Because of

Table 4

Percentage of population covered by social security[a]

	Year		
Country	1966	1968	1970
Colombia	6.21	6.22	6.21
Peru	8.90	8.90	9.00
El Salvador	4.80	4.90	4.90

[a] Source, Inter-America Institute of Social Security, Mexico City, 1973.

the small percentage of the population involved, the expenditures per capita in the social security sector and within social security in the health services, are proportionately very high indeed. Table 5 shows the expenditures per capita in the three sectors in different countries, underlining the social priorities in those societies.

Private and social security cover not more than 25 per cent of the population while consuming over 60 per cent of all health expenditures, while 70 per cent of the population consumes under 40 per cent of all expenditures (48). Since 80 per cent of all expenditures are for human resources, one could postulate that the majority of human resources follows an equal maldistribution pattern.

This distribution of resources in the health sector parallels the distribution of other resources in the tertiary and secondary sectors of the economy. Thus, social security covers a small group, the "aristocratic" portion of the labor force, and this is a group that, although not the most dynamic in the overall development, is needed to sustain the industries and services of the consumer-oriented lumpenbourgeoisie and their foreign counterparts. In addition, not unlike the use made of the social security mechanism in developed societies, social security in Latin America has been used to try to integrate (and some may say co-opt) sectors of the labor force into the "market-urban-based" economy (58).

Conclusion

The highly skewed distribution of human health resources in Latin America is a symptom of the maldistribution of resources in the different sectors of the economy, a maldistribution that, as postulated in this article, is due to the economic and cultural dependency of Latin American countries and to the control of the distribution of economic and social resources (including health resources) in those countries by a national lumpenbourgeoisie with links with foreign counterparts.

If the analyses reflected in this paper are accurate, the implications for Latin America would be quite substantial. It can be postulated that it would be unhistorical to expect that changes towards equity can occur in the present distribution of resources, within and outside the health sector, without changing the economic and cultural dependency and the control by the defined social classes of the mechanisms of control and distribution of those resources.

Indeed, in Latin America today, it would be inaccurate to expect a more equitable distribution of human health resources within a highly

Table 5

Estimated per capita expenditures by sector in selected Latin American countries[a,b]

Country	Year	Government		Social Security		Private	
		Population	Per Capita Expenditures	Population	Per Capita Expenditures	Population	Per Capita Expenditures
		%	U.S.$	%	U.S.$	%	U.S.$
Chile[c]	1968	78.6	22.80	—	—	10.8	±100
Colombia[d]	1970	85.0	9.14	6.0	27.27	9.0	⩾100
Peru[e]	1969	73.3	8.14	8.8	52.76	12.0	⩾100
El Salvador[f]	1970	84.2	5.23	4.8	35.51	11.0	⩾100

[a] Source, reference 48.

[b] Studies of private expenditures have only been carried out in Chile. We have estimated that the per capita expenditures in the other Latin American countries are at least equal to the Chilean figures since every country has a greater percentage of beds in the private sector. For Peru in 1964, the public sector accounted for 76 per cent of the total health expenditures (Hall, T. Health and Manpower in Chile. Johns Hopkins Press, Baltimore, 1971). If we assume that in 1969, 24 per cent of the expenditures were still in the private sector, this would give a per capita expenditure of U.S. $88.37 for the beneficiaries of the private sector.

[c] Source, Study of Human Resources, Chilean Ministry of Public Health, Santiago, 1970. Chile has had a national health service since 1952, accounting for 75 per cent of outpatient visits and 91 per cent of hospitalizations in the country. We have considered as beneficiaries the 78.6 per cent of the population who appeared to belong to the group having a per capita income below .59 SV (vital salary). We have assumed the 10.8 per cent of the population belonging to the group having a per capita income above 1.0 SV to be the beneficiaries in the private sector.

[d] Source, Quadrennial Projections: Colombia, 1971. Pan American Health Organization, Washington, D.C., 1971. Social Security includes the groups of Instituto Colombiano de Seguros Sociales and Caza Nacional de Prevision. According to the study on health manpower and medical education in Colombia (see reference 3), the per capita expenditures for general population in 1961–1965 were 6–10 times lower than the per capita expenditures of the "special population," which included social security for workers and employees and health services of the military forces.

[e] Source, Quadrennial Projections: Peru, 1971, Pan American Health Organization, Washington, D.C., 1971. In Peru, 22 per cent of the total population lacks any type of health service. The 73.3 per cent figure for the government sector includes this 22 per cent. Social Security includes the systems for both workers and employees.

[f] Source, Quadrennial Projections: El Salvador, 1971, Pan American Health Organization, Washington, D.C., 1971. Social Security refers to the group of the Instituto Salvadoreno de Seguridad Social.

inequitable distribution of all resources, because of the highly skewed distribution of the mechanisms of economic and political control. As King (59) and I, myself (60), have both indicated, Cuba shows that in the world of underdevelopment, an egalitarian society is required in order to achieve an equitable distribution of human health resources. To achieve it, the two parameters of underdevelopment, (a) economic and cultural dependency and (b) economic and political control by the lumpen-bourgeoisie and its foreign counterparts, have to be redefined and discontinued.

Again, if my analysis of the underdevelopment of human health resources is accurate, it would seem that the institutionalized political channels currently controlled by these groups are not adequate nor sufficient to stimulate the redistribution of resources in most of Latin America.

It is apparent that the institutionalization of the distribution of power and control in the mechanism of distribution of resources, inside as well as outside the health sector, is a profound, almost insurmountable, obstacle to the equitable distribution of human health resources. Meanwhile, as Myrdal (61) has said, the institutionalization of that power means that:

> In the Latin American situation gross violence is . . . exerted all the time, mostly against poor people to keep them suppressed. The whole economic and social order . . . must rightly be seen as "institutionalized violence."

And when the disenfranchised majority rebels against that institutionalized violence, as happened in Cuba, almost universal revulsion is expressed by the organs of communication (which are controlled by the groups that also control those structures). As Moore (62) has pointed out:

> The way nearly all history has been written imposes an overwhelming bias against revolutionary violence. . . . the use of force by the oppressed against their former masters has been the object of nearly universal condemnation. Meanwhile the day-to-day repression of "normal" society hovers dimly in the background of most history books.

And, meanwhile, the institutionalized violence continues. And when the privileges of the lumpenbourgeoisie and its international counterparts and corresponding middle classes are threatened, the implied violence in those institutional structures appears explicit, as the tragic event of this morning in Chile shows, with the brute use of the armed forces. (This paper was presented on September 11, 1973, a sad day for Latin America, when a military junta deposed the Popular Unity Government of Chile.)

Nevertheless, the persistence of that distribution of power, the main cause of the present maldistribution of resources within and outside the health sector, cannot be considered as insurmountable. Indeed, a stimulus and cause for the dissolution of that obstacle will certainly be the increasing awareness of the disenfranchised majorities of alternative patterns for the distribution of those resources and alternative strategies for determining change.

References

1. Myrdal, G. Diplomacy by terminology, Appendix I. In *Asian Drama,* Vol. 3, p. 1839, Pantheon Books, New York, 1968.

2. Ruderman, A.P. Book Review of Bryant, J. *Health and the Developing World.* in *Int. J. Health Serv.* 1(3): 293-303, 1971.

3. Social Science and Health Planning: Culture, Disease and Health Services in Colombia. Special Issue of *Milbank Mem. Fund Q.* 46(2, Part 2), 1968.

4. Kuznets, S. Quantitative aspects of the economic growth of nations. *Economic Development and Cultural Change* 11(2, Part 2), January 1963.

5. Birnbaum, N. *Toward a Critical Sociology.* Oxford University Press, New York, 1971.

6. Mills, C.W. *Sociology and Pragmatism: The Higher Learning in America.* Oxford University Press, New York, 1966.

7. Bell, D. *End of Ideology.* The Free Press, New York, 1960.

8. Blackburn, R., editor. *Ideology in Social Science.* John M. Fontana, New York, 1972.

9. Barkhuus, A., and Vargas, R. *Socio-Economic Planning in Latin America.* Pan American Health Organization, Washington, D.C., 1971 (mimeographed).

10. Parsons, T. *Structure and Process in Modern Societies.* The Free Press, New York, 1960.

11. Hoselitz, B.F. *Sociological Factors in Economic Development.* The Free Press, New York, 1960.

12. Frank, A.G. Sociology of development and underdevelopment of sociology. In Cockroft, J.D., Frank, A.G., and Johnson, D.L. *Dependence and Underdevelopment: Latin America's Political Economy,* pp. 321-397. Doubleday and Company, New York, 1972.

13. Kahn, H., and Weiner, A.J. The next 33 years. *Daedalus* pp. 705-732, Summer 1967.

14. Russett, B. *Comparado de Indicadores Sociales y Politicos.* Euramerica, S.A., 1968.

15. Mussaff, H. *The 1975-85 National Health Plan of the U.A.R.* United Arab Republic, Ministry of Health, Cairo, 1972. (mimeographed).

16. Rostow, W.W. *The Stages of Economic Growth.* Cambridge University Press, Cambridge, 1962.

17. Rostow, W.W. *The Stages of Economic Growth,* pp. 4, 7, 39. Cambridge University Press, Cambridge, 1962. Quoted in Frank, A.G. *Latin America: Underdevelopment or Revolution,* p. 40. Monthly Review Press, New York and London, 1969.

18. Frank, A.G. *Lumpenbourgeoisie: Lumpendevelopment. Dependence, Class, and Politics in Latin America.* Monthly Review Press, New York and London, 1973.

19. Baran, P. *The Longer-View: Essays Towards a Critique of Political Economy.* Monthly Review Press, New York and London, 1969.

20. Griffin, K. *Underdevelopment in Spanish America.* The MIT Press, Cambridge, Massachusetts, 1969.

21. Frank, A.G. *Latin America: Underdevelopment or Revolution.* Monthly Review Press, New York and London, 1969.

22. UNESCO Report. Cited in *New York Times,* p. 4, June 14, 1973.

23. UNESCO Report. Cited in Myrdal, G., *The Challenge of World Poverty.* Pantheon Books, New York, 1970.

24. Garcia, C. *La Educación Médica en la America Latina.* Pan American Health Organization, Washington, D.C., 1973.

25. McKeown, T. A historical appraisal of the medical task. In McLachlan, G., and McKeown, T. *Medical History and Medical Care.* Oxford University Press, New York, 1971.

26. Navarro, V. Report of a Visit to Cali. Department of Medical Care and Hospitals, School of Hygiene and Public Health, The Johns Hopkins University, 1970 (mimeographed).

27. Fucaraccio, A. Birth control and the argument of saving and investment. *Int. J. Health Serv.* 3(2): 133-144, 1973.

28. Illich, I. Outwitting the "developed" nations. In *National Health Care,* edited by R.H. Elling, pp. 263-276. Aldine Atherton, Inc., Chicago, 1971.

29. Technology and Development for Whom? *Bulletin of the Scientists and Engineers for Social Action* July 1973.

30. Navarro, V. Report of a Visit to the Planning Office of the Colombian Government. Department of Medical Care and Hospitals, School of Hygiene and Public Health, The Johns Hopkins University, 1970 (mimeographed).

31. International Development Bank. *Socio-Economic Progress in Latin America,* Eighth Annual Report. World Bank, Washington, D.C., 1968.

32. Foreign Ministries of Latin America, Declaration. Viña del Mar, Chile, 1969.

33. *Newsweek,* June 23, 1969.

34. *New York Times Magazine,* p. 79, September 16, 1973.

35. Williams, K.N., and Lockett, B.A. Migration of Foreign Physicians to the United States. Paper presented at the Pan American Conference on Health Manpower Planning, Ottawa, Canada, September 10-14, 1973 (mimeographed).

36. Ozlak, O., and Caputo, D. The Migration of Medical Personnel from Latin America to the United States: Toward an Alternative Interpretation. Paper presented at the Pan American Conference on Health Manpower Planning, Ottawa, Canada, September 10-14, 1973 (mimeographed).

37. Stevens, R., and Vermeulen, T. *Foreign Trained Physicians and American Medicine.* U.S. Department of Health, Education, and Welfare Publication No. (NIH) 73-325. U.S. Government Printing Office, Washington, D.C., 1973.

38. U.S. Foreign Assistance Program, Annual Report to Congress, 1971. U.S. Government Printing Office, Washington, D.C., 1971.

39. Basin, M. Science, Technology and the People of Latin America. Unpublished paper, 1972.

40. United Nations Economic Council for Latin America. *Economic Survey of Latin America, 1968. Part I, Some Aspects of the Latin American Economy Towards the End of the 1960s,* p. 71. E/CN.12/825. United Nations, New York, 1968. Quoted in Frank A.G. *Lumpenbourgeoisie: Lumpendevelopment. Dependence, Class, and Politics in Latin America,* p. 103. Monthly Review Press, New York and London, 1973.

41. United Nations Economic Council for Latin America. *Mobilization of Internal Resources,* p. 64. E/CN.12/827. United Nations, New York, 1970. Quoted in Frank, A. G. *Lumpenbourgeoisie: Lumpendevelopment. Dependence, Class, and Politics in Latin America,* p. 104. Monthly Review Press, New York and London, 1973.

42. Prebisch, R. *Latin American Integration.* Fondo de Cultura Economica. Mexico City, 1969 (in Spanish).

43. Peña, M. Industrialization and the national bourgeoisie. *Fichas* June 1965.

44. Petras, J. *Politics and Social Structure in Latin America.* Monthly Review Press, New York and London, 1970.

45. Marcuse, H. Repressive tolerance. In *A Critique of Pure Tolerance,* edited by R.P. Wolff, B. Moore, and H. Marcuse, pp. 81-123. Beacon Press, Boston, 1965.

46. United Nations Economic Council for Latin America. *Social Change and Social Development Policy in Latin America,* p. 79. E/CN.12/826. United Nations, New York, 1970. Quoted in Frank, A.G. *Lumpenbourgeoisie: Lumpendevelopment. Dependence, Class, and Politics in Latin America,* p. 134. Monthly Review Press, New York and London, 1973.

47. Kolko, G. *Wealth and Power in America.* Praeger Publishers, New York, 1968.

48. Navarro, V. An Analysis of Cost and Expenditures in Latin America for the Period 1965-1970. Unpublished manuscript.

49. Anderson, O.W. *Health Care: Can There Be Equity?* John Wiley and Sons, New York, 1973.

50. Bettelheim, C. Reply to A. Emmanuel, Appendix I. In Emmanuel, A. *Unequal Exchange; A Study of the Imperialism of Trade,* pp. 271-322. Monthly Review Press, New York and London, 1972.

51. de Ahumada, J. Quoted in Illich, I. Outwitting the "developed" nations. In *National Health Care,* edited by R.H. Elling, p. 266. Aldine Atherton, Inc., Chicago, 1971.

52. Godelier, M. *Rationality and Irrationality in Economics.* Monthly Review Press, New York and London, 1973.

53. Freidson, E. *Professional Dominance: The Social Structure of Medical Care.* Atherton Press, New York, 1970.

54. Miliband, R. *The State in Capitalist Society: An Analysis of the System of Power.* Weidenfeld and Nicolson, London, 1970.

55. Roemer, M. Social security for medical care: Is it justified in developing countries? *Int. J. Health Serv.* 1(4): 354-361, 1971.

56. United Nations Economic Council for Latin America. *Industrial Development in Latin America,* p. 10. E/CN.12/830. United Nations, New York, New York, 1970. Quoted in Frank, A.G. *Lumpenbourgeoisie: Lumpendevelopment. Dependence, Class, and Politics in Latin America,* p. 93. Monthly Review Press, New York and London, 1973.

57. Feder, E. *The Rape of the Peasantry: Latin America's Landholding System.* Anchor Books, Doubleday and Company, New York, 1971.

58. Rimlinger, G.V. *Welfare Policy and Industrialization in Europe, America, and Russia.* John Wiley and Sons, Inc., New York, 1971.

59. King, M. Reply to Book Review by A.P. Ruderman of Bryant, J. *Health and the Developing World.* In *Int. J. Health Serv.* 1(4): 415-416, 1971.

60. Navarro, V. Health services in Cuba: An initial appraisal. *N. Engl J. Med.* 287: 954-959, 1972.

61. Myrdal, G. *The Challenge of World Poverty,* pp. 483-484. Pantheon Books, New York, 1970.

62. Moore, B. *Social Origins of Dictatorship and Democracy: Lord and Peasant in the Making of the Modern World.* Beacon Press, Boston, 1966.

Allende's Chile:
A Case Study in the
Breaking with Underdevelopment

To all those in Chile and in the rest of Latin America who are persecuted because they believe that the way to break with the underdevelopment of health is to break with the sickness of underdevelopment.

On September 11, 1973, at nine o'clock in the morning, two battalions of infantry surrounded the Chilean presidential palace in Santiago. From ten o'clock until two o'clock, the troops bombarded the building, killing most of the staff, including the President of Chile, Salvador Allende.[1] Just a few yards from the palace can be found the most luxurious hotel in Santiago, the Careras Hotel, which is owned by the U.S. Sheraton chain. The New York *Times* correspondent in the city reported that in that hotel, as in very many places at that time in Chile, the maids, cleaners, and blue-collar workers gathered in the basement in fear and anger over the fall of what they considered their government. Up on the top floor, meanwhile, the hotel manager invited his patrons to drink champagne with him, to celebrate the mililary coup and the fall of the Unidad Popular government. Not very far away, in the Medical College building, the Chilean Medical Association sent a telegram of support for the coup (3). Meanwhile, in most health centers and hospitals, and in most working class and rural communities, the health workers, the blue-collar workers, the low-income peasantry, the unemployed, and the poor, that sector of the Chilean population that Neruda had defined as the "disenfranchised majorities," were presenting resistance to the military takeover. The strength of the resistance is evidenced by the fact that today, ten months after that morning in September, the country is still in a state of siege. And the military has had to establish a repression defined by the correspondent of *Le Monde* in Santiago as "the carnage of the working class and of the poor" (4, p. 12). Thousands of miles away, according to the Washington correspondent of *Le Monde Diplomatique,* the atmos-

---

[1]For an accurate report of the events that took place during and after the coup, see the dispatches from Santiago by the correspondents of the Washington *Post* and *Le Monde,* and by J. Kandell (1) of the New York *Times.* The Santiago correspondents of the *Wall Street Journal* are notoriously inaccurate. For an excellent detailed critique of the misinformation provided by the *Wall Street Journal,* see Birns (2).

phere in the "corporate corridors of power in Washington was one of cautious delight, with some embarrassment" (4).

Why all these events? How were they linked? And more important, what is the meaning of those events in Chile for Latin America as a whole at the present time?

In this presentation I will try to give you my perception of what happened to Chile's health sector and why it happened. And I will attempt some tentative conclusions. Also, and since it is my assumption that the health sector in any society mirrors the rest of that society, I will try to describe the evolution of Chile's health services within the overall parameters that define the general underdevelopment of Chile.

By Way of Introduction

In order to explain the events in Chile, both within as well as outside the health sector, we should first look at the causes of underdevelopment in Chile, which, as I have postulated in the preceding article (5), are the same determinants that shape the structure, function, and distribution of resources in the health sector. And before beginning this discussion, it may be helpful to briefly reiterate some of the conclusions that were reached in that article.

Indeed, the causes of underdevelopment, not only in Chile, but also in most of Latin America, are not due (as is believed in most of the leading circles of government and academia of developed countries and in the international agencies) to (a) the scarcity of the proper "values" and technology in the poor countries, (b) the scarcity of capital and resources, and (c) the insufficient diffusion of capital, values, and technology from the developed societies to the cities of the underdeveloped countries and from there to the rural areas. Quite the opposite of that interpretation of underdevelopment, the causes of underdevelopment are precisely the existence in Chile, as well as in the rest of Latin America, of those "conditions of development"—that is, (a) too much cultural and technological dependency on the developed countries, and (b) the underuse and improper use of the existing capital by the lumpenbourgeoisie and its foreign counterparts.

Actually, the highly skewed distribution of both economic and political power in Chile, with control of that underused and improperly used capital by the national bourgeoisie and its foreign counterparts, is at the roots of Chile's underdevelopment.

To understand the underdevelopment of health resources in Chile, then, we have to start with a description of the skewed distribution of economic and political power between the different classes in Chile. And, although each class contains different groups with different interests, there is still a certain uniformity of political and economic behavior within each class which allows us to break Chilean society into basically three classes.[2]

At the top, we have 10 per cent of the population, who control 60 per cent of the wealth (income and property) of that society, and who determine the patterns of investment, production, and consumption in Chilean society. Because their economic, political, and social power, however, is dependent on the power of the bourgeoisie of the developed countries, Frank (7) adds the expression "lumpen" to the term bourgeoisie. Dependent on the lumpenbourgeoisie are the middle classes. Far from being a progressive force, as the middle classes were in the developed societies following the industrial revolution, the middle classes in Latin America were and are a mere economic appendage to the lumpenbourgeoisie.

Below these two classes is the majority of the population, the blue-collar workers, the peasantry, the unemployed, and the poor, representing 65 per cent of the Chilean population and owning only 12 per cent of the wealth of that society (8).[3]

The Structure of Health Services in Chile

Not unexpectedly, the class structure of Chile is replicated in its health services. Thus, the governmental health service or National Health

[2]The upper class includes the monopolistic bourgeoisie, the large agrarian bourgeoisie, the large landowners, the large urban non-monopolistic bourgeoisie, and the small and medium urban bourgeoisie. The middle class includes the petite bourgeoisie, the professionals, the white collars, state civil servants, and large sectors of the middle echelons of the armed forces. The working class includes the workers in monopolistic and large industries (the best organized and most politicized workers in Chile), the workers in small and medium-sized industries, and the subproletariat. The peasantry includes the farm workers and sharecroppers. For an excellent description of each class, see the Popular Action Unity Movement (MAPU) pamphlet, "The Character of the Chilean Revolution," published as Chapter 10 in Johnson (6).

[3]In terms of income distribution, in the 1960s this was as follows: "Five per cent of the population, composed mainly of urban owners of capital, receives 40 per cent of national income; twenty per cent of the population, mainly urban employees, receives 40 per cent of national income; fifty per cent of the population, mainly urban workers in industry and trade, receives 15 per cent of national income; and twenty-five per cent of the population, mainly rural agricultural workers, receives 5 per cent of national income" Frank (9, p. 106).

Service (NHS) covers the working class, peasantry, the unemployed, and the poor—groups which, together with a small fraction of the lowest-paid white-collar workers also covered by the NHS, represent approximately 70 per cent of the Chilean population; voluntary health insurance (SERMENA) covers the middle class, who represent approximately 22 per cent of the Chilean people; and the fee-for-service, out-of-pocket, "market" medicine covers the lumpenbourgeoisie, approximately 8 per cent of Chileans. And, again, not unexpectedly, expenditures per capita are lowest in the government sector, higher in the insurance sector, and much larger in the private sector. Actually, expenditure figures show that the top two groups, the lumpenbourgeoisie and middle classes, while representing 30 per cent of the Chilean population, consumed 60 per cent of Chile's health expenditures in the time period from 1968 to 1969, while the working class, peasantry, unemployed, and poor, representing 70 per cent of the population, consumed only 40 per cent of those national health expenditures (10, p. 93, 183 and 186). Moreover, and reflecting the increasing income differential between the upper and lower classes, those differences of consumption have been increasing, not decreasing. Indeed, while private sector consumption in 1958 represented 41 per cent of the national health expenditures, by 1963 that percentage had grown to 57 per cent, and by 1968 to 60 per cent (11, p. 10). Thus, the private sector of consumption increased from 2.0 per cent of the gross national product in 1960 to 3.7 per cent in 1968, while public sector consumption actually decreased from 3.2 per cent in 1960 to 2.5 per cent in 1968. This expansion in private sector health consumption was due primarily to increased consumption per capita in the private sector, since the percentage of the population in both the lumpenbourgeoisie and middle classes has remained practically the same (8). In summary, then, the distribution and consumption of health resources in Chile reflects Chile's class distribution, and this leads to a situation in which family expenditures for health services in the lower classes are a tenth of the amount spent by the upper classes (12).

However, as important as the knowledge of the present distribution of resources in the health sector may be, it might be still more important to know how this distribution of resources, reflected in the class system, came about. Actually, it is worth noting that, while in the evolution of the Chilean health services we find some elements that are unique to the Chilean situation, there are also quite a number of characteristics which are similar to those seen in other countries, including our own. (For a succinct review of the main historical events in Chile during this century, see Scientists and Engineers for Social and Political Action, reference 13.)

The concept of health care as a basic right was accepted in Chile as far back as 1925, when it was written into the Chilean Constitution that health is a human right and that the state has the responsibility of guaranteeing health care for its citizens. The gap between theory and practice was a wide one, however, and it was not until 1952 that a National Health Service was established, initially to take care of the blue-collar workers, and then, in successive stages, other sectors of the population such as the peasantry, the unemployed, and the poor.[4] There are several reasons, as many as there are theories, for the creation of the National Health Service at that time. One reason is the situation of the Chilean economy in the thirties and forties. In the Depression which hit the world economy in the thirties, international demand for raw materials and primary products fell off markedly, creating a major crisis in dependent economies such as Chile's, where the main exports were those goods. It was not until the forties, during World War II, that the demand for Chile's products, and primarily for copper, Chile's main export, began to revive. It was at this time that the lumpenbourgeoisie and its foreign counterparts saw an opportunity to develop the sluggish economy according to their own schemes, with industrialization as the main stimulation for that development. Because they wanted to build up the economy, it was to their advantage to have a healthy work force, particularly in the industrial sector. In fact, a major aim of the National Health Service was to "produce a healthy and productive labor force" (11, p. 12) and the statutory law establishing the National Health Service actually states that a prime objective of the Service is to "guide the development of the child and the young, and the maintenance of the adult for their full capacity as future and present producers" (14).

The intended industrialization of the country required great sacrifices and, as has occurred in most countries, the burden of these sacrifices fell not on upper but on lower class shoulders. It was during the decade 1940–1950 that a large regressive distribution of income took place at the expense of the lower-income groups. Wages during that period fell from 27 to 21 per cent of the national income, and the economic gap between the classes increased dramatically. These developments were accompanied by great repression, with the intent to destroy the working-class-based parties. Not surprisingly, this period of Chilean history was marked by worker and peasant uprisings, and great social

[4]Before 1952, the labor insurance and the welfare systems were in charge of the care of the blue-collar workers (although not the workers' families) and the poor.

unrest. And the threatened lumpenbourgeoisie responded to this not only with repression but with social legislation. This reaction was not unlike that of Bismarck during the previous century in Germany, with, besides repression, the creation of social security and the founding of a National Health Insurance scheme to care for the blue-collar workers, and later the peasantry, unemployed, and poor. The intent of these changes was to co-opt the unsettling forces. But the concession of one class was the gain of the other. Naturally the working-class-based parties not only supported but fought for the creation of the National Health Service. And it was none other than the late President Allende, at that time a member of the Chilean Senate for the Socialist Party, who introduced and sponsored the law establishing the National Health Service.

In that respect the Chilean experience in the 1950s repeated the experience with social security in other countries. Indeed, here let me quote Sigerist, that great medical historian and professor of medical history at Johns Hopkins back in the 1940s. I believe his words, spoken in his Heath Clark Lectures at the London School of Hygiene, the same year—1952—that the National Health Service was created in Chile, are relevant not only to the Chilean situation of the 1950s but also to our present debate on national health insurance here in the United States (15; also quoted in 16, p. 317).

> Social-security legislation came in waves and followed a certain pattern. Increased industrialization created the need; strong political parties representing the interests of the workers seemed a potential threat to the existing order, or at least to the traditional system of production, and an acute scare such as that created by the French Commune stirred Conservatives into action and social-security legislation was enacted. In England at the beginning of our century the second industrial revolution was very strongly felt. The Labour Party entered parliament and from a two-party country England developed into a three-party country. The Russian revolution of 1905 was suppressed to be sure, but seemed a dress rehearsal for other revolutions to follow. Social legislation was enacted not by the Socialists but by Lloyd George and Churchill. A third wave followed World War I when again the industries of every warfaring country were greatly expanded, when, as a result of the war, the Socialist parties grew stronger everywhere, and the Russian revolution of 1917 created a red scare from which many countries are still suffering. Again social-security legislation was enacted in a number of countries.

> Every historical pattern we set up is to a certain extent artificial and history never repeats itself unaltered. But patterns are useful because they help us to understand conditions. When we look at the American scene we find the

need for health insurance and a red scare that could not be stronger, but America has no Socialist party, no politically active labour movement that could bring pressure upon the Government. The existing order is not threatened from any side and conservative parties do not feel the need for action on these lines.

How applicable this quotation is to our present situation in the United States is for you to decide. As for its applicability to the Chilean situation in the 1950s, it is clear that the creation of social security and the National Health Service was also a response by the right to claims and threats from the left.

The middle and upper classes continued in the private sector on a fee-for-service, direct payment to physicians basis, following the market model in which health services are sold and bought like any other commodity.

The attitude of the medical profession toward the National Health Service has been ambivalent. On the one side, it needs it, since the consumer power for the majority of the population covered by the National Health Service was, and continues to be, very low indeed. And the National Health Service has always been an important source of income for the 90 per cent of Chile's physicians who work for it either on a part- or full-time basis (11).

On the other hand, the medical profession maintained profound reservations about the National Health Service because it feared government intervention. This explains why, as its conditions of acceptance of the service, it asked (a) that the Chilean Medical Association be appointed, by law, as the watchdog of the National Health Service, to defend the economic and other interests of the medical profession, and (b) that there still be private practice, on a fee-for-service basis, for private patients, who would be able to use National Health Service facilities.[5]

It was not until the 1960s, when an economic depression hit Chile and the costs of health care increased, that both the consuming middle classes on the one side, and the physicians on the other, began a movement that led to the creation in 1968 of a health insurance plan (SERMENA) similar to our Blue Cross-Blue Shield, to cover both

[5]Full-time physicians working for the National Health Service are supposed to work, in theory, six hours a day, being paid on a salary basis. The arrangements for the part-time physicians are similar to those in the National Health Service in Britain, with privileges for "amenity beds" for the physicians' private clientele within the National Health Service hospitals.

hospitalization and ambulatory care, with maintenance of the fee-for-service payment to the physicians. As with our Blues, the creation of SERMENA was very much a result of concern by the providers that the increasing costs of medical care were threatening to force their private clientele out of the market. The Frei administration, whose main constituency was the middle classes, approved and stimulated the creation of this insurance, which covers the majority of professionals, small owners, petite bourgeoisie, and white-collar workers.

With the establishment of SERMENA, then, the Chilean class structure was formalized and replicated within the health sector, with the National Health Service taking care of 70 per cent or the majority of the population—the blue collar workers, peasants, unemployed, and poor—and the health insurance scheme (SERMENA) taking care of the middle classes (20 per cent) and increasing sectors of the lumpenbourgeoisie (2 per cent). (For a historical review of the health services in Chile, see references 17 and 18. Both articles are in Spanish.)

The Distribution of Resources by Regions

Related to this maldistribution of resources by social class, there is a maldistribution of resources by regions, depending on whether the areas are urban or rural. Chile, a long, narrow country that is 2,600 miles in length, is 75 per cent urban and 25 per cent rural, and 30 per cent of the population lives in the capital, Santiago. Analyzing the distribution of resources, we find that the number of visits per annum per capita in Santiago (three) is twice that of the rural areas, while the personal expenditures for health services in Santiago ($38) are over four times those in the rural areas ($9), for both ambulatory and hospital care. (For an excellent review of the distribution of health resources in the National Health Service in Chile, see reference 19.)

Santiago, although it only has a third of the Chilean population, also has 60 per cent of all physicians and 50 per cent of all dentists. In terms of environmental services, 80 per cent of the water supply and 65 per cent of the sewerage system is considered adequate in the urban areas, compared with only 20 per cent and 9 per cent, respectively, in the rural ones (20).

As I have explained in the preceding article (5), these rural areas are not marginal areas that the modern sector has not reached. In fact, quite the contrary, their poverty is due to their link to the modern sector, and the wealth of the urban areas is partially based on the poverty of the rural ones. However dramatic this statement may sound, the evidence shows that a significant part of the wealth of the urban-based lumpenbourgeoisie comes primarily from the extractive industries and agriculture, which are situated where most of the poverty in Chile is—in the rural areas. (For a detailed and excellent explanation of this argument, see reference 9, pp. 1–20.)

Why This Maldistribution?

In the paper referred to earlier (5), I attempted to analyze some of the reasons for this maldistribution, which are rather typical of most Latin American countries. And, as I indicated earlier, we cannot understand the maldistribution of resources in the health sector without analyzing the distribution of economic and political power in these societies, i.e., the question of who controls what and whom, or, as it is usually phrased in political economy, who controls the means of production and reproduction?

In Chile, as in most Latin American countries, the lumpenbourgeoisie controls most of the wealth, property, and income in the society. Thus, they are the ones who do most of the saving, who direct the investments and greatly influence the different affairs of state, and who primarily control the workings of the executive, legislative, judicial, and military arms of government. Above all, they control the distribution of resources in the primary, secondary, and tertiary sectors of the economy. In the tertiary sector, they influence the distribution of resources in the health sector by (a) expounding the "market model" system of allocating resources, whereby resources are distributed according to consuming rather than producing power, i.e., upper class, urban-based consumer power; (b) influencing the means of reproduction, i.e. urban-based medical education; and (c) controlling the social content and nature of the medical profession, as a result of the unavailability and inaccessibility of university education to the majority of the population. Actually, the medical students come primarily from the professional and lumpenbourgeoisie classes, which represent less than 12 per cent of the Chilean population. Let me illustrate this point with figures on the father's occupations of the 264 first-year students in the School of Medicine of the University of Chile in 1971: managers and professionals (70.4 per cent); white-collar workers (16.0 per cent); blue-collar (4.1 per cent); and others (9.5 per cent). The category "others," incidentally, does not include peasants. The peasantry, 30 per cent of the labor force, had not a son or a daughter in the main medical school of Chile (21, p. 4).

Another mechanism of control used by the lumpenbourgeoisie in the health sector is its influence, tantamount to control, over the highly centralized, urban-based state organs, so that the public sector, controlled by the different branches of the state, is made to serve its needs. Until 1970 the executive, legislative, and judicial branches were all controlled by those political parties that represent the lumpenbourgeoisie and the middle classes. In the election of 1970, however, the executive, though not the other branches of the state, changed hands and passed partially into the control of the working-class-based parties. (For a detailed explanation of this point, see the series of articles edited by Cockcroft et al, reference 22, Part II.)

Consequences of this Control: The Priorities in the Health Sector

This control by the bourgeoisie of the means of production in the health sector leads to a pattern of production aimed primarily at the satisfaction of the bourgeoisie's pattern of consumption. And this pattern of consumption of the lumpenbourgeoisie, the setters of tastes and values of these societies, mimics the pattern of consumption of the bourgeoisie of the developed countries.

Not surprisingly, then, we find a pattern of production in the health services of Chile that is very similar to the pattern of production in most health services of developed countries, i.e. a system of health services that is highly oriented toward (a) specialized, hospital-based medicine as opposed to community medicine; (b) urban, technologically-intensive medicine in contrast to rural, labor-intensive medicine; (c) curative medicine as different from preventive medicine; and (d) personal health services as opposed to environmental health services. Needless to say, considering the type of health problems prevalent in Chile, where malnutrition and infectious diseases are the main causes of mortality and morbidity, the best strategy to combat the problems which affect the majority would be to emphasize precisely the opposite patterns of production to those currently prevalent in the health sector. This would imply emphasis on rural, labor-intensive, and community-oriented medicine, while giving far greater priority to the preventive and environmental health services than to personal health and curative services.

This mimical behavior of the lumpenbourgeoisie is explained by its interest in having the "latest" in medicine, with a concomitant growth of open-heart surgery units, coronary care units, organ transplants, and the like, representing the "Cadillacs" or "Rolls Royces" of medicine, an order of medical priorities that is bad enough in developed countries and even worse in developing ones. Indeed, this order of priorities diverts much needed resources from the production of health services aimed at the care not of the few, but of the many.

Control by the few of the production of health resources also determines a pattern of reproduction in Chile's medical education that leads to a distribution of specialties which follows very closely, by types and percentages of specialties, that in the developed countries. Table 1 shows the percentage distribution of physicians in certain specialties. You

Table 1

Percentage Distribution of Physicians by Some Specialties

Country	Year	General Practice	Public Health	Surgery	Pediatrics
Chile	1972	14.0	3.2	18.2	10.0
United States	1970	17.8	0.8	20.0	6.0

Source: Adapted from Department of Human Resources, Pan American Health Organization. *Health Manpower in the Americas,* Washington, D.C., 1973.

can see that surgery, for example, the typical technological, hospital-based specialty, represents the top specialty by percentage of physicians, with pediatrics and public health being the lowest categories. It should be obvious that in a country with 38 per cent of the population under 15 years of age, and with a type of morbidity caused by environmental and nutritional deficiencies, there is an oversupply of the former and an undersupply of the latter.

Table 2 shows that expenditures per capita on environmental health services are a very small fraction of total expenditures in the health sector, with the majority of resources going to curative services and the largest percentage to hospitals. The well known economist de Ahumada (23), Navarro (5), and very many others (see Navarro and Ruderman, 24) have emphasized that the health services required for a developing country are services that are not technological but labor-intensive, not hospital- but community-oriented, not curative but preventive, and aimed not at personal but environmental health services. This suggested order of priorities is precisely opposite to the one followed in Chile and in the

Table 2

Estimated Expenditures of the Chilean Health Sector
in Medical Care and Water and Sewerage Supply
Per Capita and by Percentages of Total
Health Expenditure, in 1969

Medical Care		Water and Sewerage	
Per Capita Expenditure (US $)	%	Per Capita Expenditure (US $)	%
24	94	1.5	6

Source: P.S. Sepulveda. *Analysis of health expenditures in Chile* (in Spanish). University of Chile, Santiago, 1972.

majority of Latin American countries, which, as I have explained, is a result of the pattern of economic and political control in those countries.

The Election of the Unidad Popular (UP) Government

Having detailed the situation before the coming of Allende's government, let me now define what a government whose main constituencies were precisely the disenfranchised blue-collar working classes and peasantry did, and intended to do, in the area of health services. As a song, popular among the upper class during the Allende administration, said (quoted in reference 25, p. 169):

> Under Alessandri [National Party], gentlemen governed,
> under Frei, the noveaux riches [and not so rich],
> and now, with Allende, govern the ragged ones.

The Unidad Popular government, which took office in 1970, was a coalition administration, a popular front government of very different parties with no one in a clear position of leadership.[6] Interparty struggles were part of the daily political scene, with cabinet positions given

[6]The parties of the coalition included the Socialist and Communist Parties, the most powerful within the coalition, the Radical Party (a lower-middle-class party), MAPU (United Popular Action Movement), and the IC (Christian Left). These two last parties were split-offs from the Christian Democratic Party (PDC), the main bourgeois party. To the left of the UP coalition parties, there were the MIR (Revolutionary Left Movement) and the PCR (Revolutionary Communist Party), two very small radical left parties which did not participate in, but supported, the UP government.

according to the relative importance of each party within that coalition. The Ministry of Public Health, not a basic post within the government (or, I would add, in most governments and in most countries), was given to a minority party, the Radical Party, whose constituency was a small sector of the middle class. The major health policies, however, were defined by the Cabinet, chaired by President Allende, with a Socialist and Communist majority. President Allende, himself, incidentally, a physician by profession, had long been acquainted with the development of the health services, both as a member of the Senate for thirty years and as the youngest Minister of Public Health during the Popular Front government in 1938. It is thus not surprising that although the distribution of health resources was not the top issue within the administration, it was not at the bottom either. Moreover, the evolution of events in the health sector did mirror the overall series of events that took place in Chilean society as a whole during the period 1970 to 1973.

The three main commitments that the Allende administration made in the health sector were the integration of the different branches of the health services (with the exception of the armed forces health service) into one health service, the democratization of the health services institutions, and the change of priorities in the health sector, placing greater emphasis on ambulatory care and preventive services. Let me start by looking at the third of these commitments and examine ambulatory and preventive services.

The Change toward More Ambulatory and Preventive Services

The National Health Service in Chile had been organized following a regional system back in 1958, during the Alessandri administration, a conservative administration that was committed to "clean" and "efficient" government. This regionalization further developed during the years of the Frei administration from 1964 to 1970, and was strengthened during Allende's time. There were three levels of care: a primary care or health center level, looking after a population of approximately 30,000 people; a secondary care or community hospital level, looking after a population of approximately a quarter to a half-million; and a tertiary care or regional center level, in charge of the care provided to a population of one to one and a half-million people.

This regionalized National Health Service during the Alessandri and Frei administrations has been characterized as being largely centralized, bureaucratic, and very hospital-oriented (20). Actually, not unlike the situation in the United Kingdom and the United States, for instance, a very large percentage of all National Health Service expenditures, close to 50 per cent, went to hospitals. The Allende administration tried to reverse these priorities by shifting the emphasis toward the health centers through the allocation of more resources to those centers. One example of this shift was that, out of the six hours a day physicians worked in the NHS, during the Allende administration at least two or the equivalent had to be spent in the health centers. Another example is that the Compulsory Community Service, whereby all physicians had to work for a period of three years in an urban or rural health center (either when their degrees were granted, or at the end of their residencies), was expanded to five years. Also, the number of hours in which the health centers were open to the community was expanded into the late hours of the evening, and, in some communities, such as Santiago, they were even open twenty-four hours a day. During the night hours, the centers were staffed with final-year medical students, under the overall supervision of available physicians (26).

Needless to say, none of these changes endeared the Allende administration to the majority of physicians. The policies were, however, very popular with the majority of the population, since they increased the accessibility of resources to the population, providing services where people lived (i.e. in the communities). Actually, following the implementation of these policies, immediately after Allende took power, one result was that there was a large increase in the consumption of ambulatory services, primarily among children. Indeed, the overall number of ambulatory visits by children increased in just the first six months of 1971 by 17 per cent over the whole country, and by 21 per cent for the city of Santiago (20, p. 11). Also, and as part of this new orientation toward the community, preventive-service activities such as immunization, vaccinations, prenatal care, and others, were emphasized. These preventive activities, incidentally, were provided not as separate programs, but as part of the usual services of the health centers. Another change, by the way, was to expand the distribution of half a liter of milk per day, previously provided to children under five, to include children up to 15 years of age.

While these activities were far from uniformly successful, they seem to have stimulated popular support and popular involvement in the delivery of health services. And this leads me to what may be considered one of the most important achievements in the health sector during the Allende administration: the democratization of the health institutions.

The Democratization of the Health Institutions

The National Health Service in Chile has been referred to as a mammoth bureaucracy that was not very responsive to the needs of the citizenry in general and to the local consumers and communities in particular. However, the increase in working-class political consciousness as a result of the continuous economic crisis of the 1960s, besides making the working class parties more powerful, also created, at the community level, a demand for popular participation in social and economic areas. This growing demand explains the creation by the Frei administration of the Community Health Councils, which were aimed at stimulating the participation of the communities in running the health institutions, either at the primary, secondary, or tertiary care levels (11). Not unlike our health advisory councils here in the United States, and the newly established district community councils in Britain, these early councils were supposed to be merely advisory to the director of the institution who was appointed by the central government.[7] The councils seem not to have been very successful as a mechanism for community participation in the health sector. They were perceived by the working class as a co-opting mechanism. Indeed, as indicated by the First Congress of the Trade Unions of Chilean Health Workers (30; also quoted in reference 11, pp 23–24):

> With community participation [equivalent to our American consumer participation], our bourgeoisie gives our workers a feeling of participation, but without an actual and authentic power of decision . . . with this policy the decisions that are taken by the bourgeoisie are legitimized by the participation of the workers, who not only don't have any power of decision, but do not have the right to complain afterwards about those decisions either, since, in theory, the workers did participate in those decisions.

It was felt that, as another writer pointed out, "community participation is an intent of co-option of the community dwellers and legitimization of the power of the bourgeoisie" (31, p. 15).

Responsive to a demand not for community participation but for community control, the Allende administration committed itself to the democratization of the health institutions, stating in its political platform dealing with the health sector that "the communities—people—are the most important resources in the health sector, both as producers and as

[7]There is voluminous literature in both the United States and the United Kingdom on consumer participation. For a representative view in the United States, see Sheps (27) and in the United Kingdom, see Weaver (28). For a description of the roles of the district community councils, see Great Britain, Ministry of Health (29).

decision makers" (32). Democratization, incidentally, took place in other areas besides the health sector, although in that sector it did go further. A likely reason for this may have been that most of the health institutions, health centers, hospitals, and the like, were already in the public sector and thus were amenable to government influence. The majority of economic institutions, on the other hand, remained during the Allende administration in the private sector.

The democratization of the health institutions took place via the executive committees, which, as their name suggests, were the executive or top administrative authorities in each institution. They had a tripartite composition, with a third of the board elected by community organizations (trade unions, Federation of Chilean Women, farmers' associations, etc.), another third elected by the workers and employees working in that institution, and one-third appointed by the local and central government authorities. Each level elected the level above itself, so that the executive committees of the health centers elected the executive committees of the community hospitals and these elected the executive committees of the regional hospitals. Their authority was limited to an overall budget for each institution, and it had to be spent within the guidelines established by the planning authorities, which were in turn accountable to the central government.

How did this democratization work? Before replying to this question, I should point out that democratization was a result of popular and community pressure on the one side and the commitment of the ruling political parties to implement it on the other. A key element for that implementation was the civil servants of the National Health Service, who mostly belonged to the opposition parties and whose outlook, like that of most civil servants in any country I know of, be it socialist or capitalist, tended to be conservative. By a large majority, 86 per cent to be precise, they were in favor of community participation but against community control (33, p. 68).

Let me explain what I mean by the conservative attitude of the civil service. Civil servants, or, as Miliband (34) defines them, the "servants of the state," tend to defend the status quo and thus tend to be in general conservative. As Crossman (35) has said for the Labour Party in Britain, and Myrdal (36) has said for the Social Democrats in Sweden, both parties have always encountered the unspoken resistance of the civil service in trying to implement their policies. And even in China, after thirty years of Communist Party rule, as the need to have a cultural revolution showed, the civil service opposed the changes advocated by powerful sectors of the ruling party (37). Chile, then, was no exception.

Needless to say, another group that did not welcome democratization of the health institutions was the medical profession, and this added to the long list of grievances that the medical profession had against the Allende adminstration. The democratization, however, proved to be quite popular among the citizens of the communities, and in a survey carried out for a doctoral thesis (33), the majority of community representatives interviewed expressed "satisfaction" to "active satisfaction" with the democratization of the institutions. And, not surprisingly, the communities' involvment with their health institutions did increase, side by side with the increased politicization of the population which was the main characteristic of the period during 1970 to 1973.

Another example of community participation was the Councils for Distribution of Food and Price Controls (JAP), neighborhood committees created by communities to avoid speculation and oversee the distribution of popular items to consumers.[8] Also, the community control movement was parallel and went hand in hand with the movement of workers' control, another commitment of the Allende administration. Indeed, in the 320 enterprises that were in the public sector during Allende's thirty-four months as President, the management in these businesses was run by an administrative council composed of five worker representatives (three blue-collar workers, one technical person, and one professional person), five state representatives, and one state-appointed administrator. Let me add something here that my business school colleagues will very likely not believe. It is that an American scholar in Chile found, in a multivariate analysis of productivity in a sample of factories, that productivity in the factories was related to participation by both workers and employees in the process of decision making. The variable of the political consciousness of the factory workers was more important in explaining increased participation and production than were other variables such as capital-labor ratio, technological complexity, technological type, or size of the vertical or horizontal integration (references 13 and 38).

All these related movements of community and worker control grew parallel to the politicization of the population and increased very rapidly after the first abortive attempt at a military coup on June 29, 1973, when, spontaneously, twenty factories were taken over and directly managed by

[8]The JAPs originated in 1971 to assist in the distribution process, making sure that local shopkeepers did not charge above the official prices and that they did not divert items to the black market (38).

both the workers and the communities. And it was in response to the first owners' strike in October 1972 that the workers themselves took over the management of the factories. As Steenland (39, p. 18) has indicated:

> The October offensive of the bourgeoisie further polarized the Chilean political scene. Every organization and almost every individual was forced to take a position for or against the government.

It was at this time that the Industrial Strife Committees were established to coordinate the management of all factories located within a vicinity or community and to set up committees within each factory in charge of production, distribution, defense, and mobilization. Also, these committees stimulated the creation at the community level of the Neighborhood Commands, broadly based community committees in charge of the coordination of the community social services, including health, and the mobilization of the population (40).

These movements of community and worker control, stimulated at first by the Allende government, grew and achieved a momentum of their own, until they expanded into the main sectors of the economy and forced a hesitant government into a defensive position. As Sweezy (41) has indicated, the government went from a leadership position to one of a follower, far behind, and hesitant to grant what was being requested and demanded in those movements. And, as both Sweezy (41) and Petras (42) point out, it was this hesitancy that seems to have partially stimulated the downfall of the Unidad Popular government.

And speaking of hesitancy, let me describe the third characteristic of the Allende government in the health sector, the one in which it showed greatest hesitation and the one that brought about the greatest opposition: the policy of ending two-class medicine, with integration of both the National Health Service and SERMENA into just one system. In the health sector, this policy was Allende's Achilles' heel.

The Intent of Creating a Classless Health Service

Allende had a commitment, as part of his political platform, to the creation of one national health service that would have integrated both the National Health Service and the voluntary health insurance of SERMENA (20). Interestingly enough, it was never intended to include within this integrated system the health services for the armed forces. Actually, a characteristic of the Allende administration was its efforts not to antagonize the military, allowing and even encouraging the granting of special privileges to those in uniform (43).[9]

How that integration of health services was to take place was not spelled out, either in the Unidad Popular platform or in subsequent policy statements once Allende was in power. Also, fearful of further antagonizing the lumpenbourgeoisie, the middle classes, and the medical profession, the UP government kept postponing the implementation of the commitment for a more propitious time.

Opposition to the integration measure was expected from the lumpenbourgeoisie and middle classes because integration could have meant the leveling off of their consumption, with the consumption of the majority of Chileans being cared for by the National Health Service. Indeed, those classes feared absorption of their health services by the National Health Service, with the resources they had always enjoyed having to be shared with the majority of the population.

The medical profession opposed integration for both professional and class reasons. Among the former reasons was the fear of losing the much desired fee-for-service and "private practice" type of medicine typical of SERMENA. In addition, it feared integration in the National Health Service would mean the loss of its independence and of its economic power. Among the class reasons was the increasing curtailment of consumption that both the lumpenbourgeoisie and the middle classes were exposed to in the Allende administration as a result of an alleged scarcity of resources both outside and within the health sector.

Since much has been written on that scarcity of resources, allow me to dwell on this point for just a moment. There is a widely held belief in some sectors of our academia and press that the cause for this scarcity of goods, commodities, and services, and even for the fall of the UP government, was the incompetence of the economic advisers to the Allende administration. As one of the representatives of this belief, Paul N. Rosenstein-Rodan (45), recently wrote in the New York *Times,* "undergraduate economic students would have known better" than the

---

[9]This policy was part of a deliberate intent by Allende to co-opt the military, which traditionally has had very strong ties with the U.S. military. It is interesting to note that in 1973, at the height of the economic blockade against Chile, Chile's armed forces remained, along with Venezuela's, the main recipients in Latin America of U.S. aid for training officers. And, when no other public agency or department within the UP government could get international loans and credit, the Chilean military received credit to buy F5E supersonic jets (40). Actually, the U.S. granted to the military in Chile a total of $45.5 million in aid during fiscal years 1971 to 1974, double the total granted in the previous four years. As Admiral Raymond Peet testified before the Senate Appropriations Committee, "One of the big advantages that accrues to the United States from such a foreign sales program is the considerable influence we derive from providing the support for these aircraft" (40 and 44).

economists advising the Chilean government. According to this interpretation of the scarcities and of the fall of Allende, other possible explanatory factors, such as the U.S.-led economic blockade, the boycott of the production of those goods and services by U.S. and Chilean economic and professional interests, and the manipulation of the international market by those interests to damage the Chilean balance of payments, are easily dismissed as mere "left wing demonologies." Actually, in the widely publicized article by Rosenstein-Rodan quoted before, these possible alternate explanatory factors are not mentioned once. And since the acceptance of the idea of "economic incompetence" absolves the powerful economic and professional groups, both internationally and in Chile, of any major responsibility for the events in Chile, this interpretation of the scarcity of resources and of the fall of Allende is the most widely held, supported, and circulated view, not only, of course, among those economic groups, but also among those sectors of the U.S. press and academia sympathetic to those groups.

Because this view is so frequently expressed both outside and within the health sector, let me then present other alternate explanations for the scarcity of goods, commodities, and services under Allende.

When the UP government took office, 47 per cent of the population was undernourished (46, p. 17), 68 per cent of the nation's workers were earning less than what was officially defined as a subsistence wage, and there was an unemployment rate of 6 per cent in Chile as a whole and a rate of 7.1 per cent in Santiago (13, pp. 14–19). The poorest 60 per cent of Chilean families received only 28 per cent of the national income, while the richest 6 per cent received 46 per cent (39, p. 9). Over one-quarter of the population of Santiago lived in flimsy shacks without running water. Meanwhile, industrial production was running at only 75 per cent capacity (39).

Just one year after the UP took office, the industrial production went up to 100 per cent capacity, unemployment went down to 3.8 per cent (5.5 per cent in Santiago), workers received a 20–30 per cent increase in real wages, and the percentage of the national income in wages went up from 51 per cent in 1970 to 60.7 per cent in 1971. Meanwhile, inflation was kept down to 22 per cent in 1971, as compared to an average 26.5 per cent in the years 1965–1970.

This dramatic increase of the purchasing power of the majority of the population and the larger availability of resources to all, not only to a few, created a great increase in the demand for goods and services, which, as I indicated before, was also reflected in the consumption of health services, primarily ambulatory health services.[10]

Because of the increase in demand for basic goods such as food, the UP government had to import more than the usual 60 per cent of food that Chile had to bring in from abroad. Indeed, Chile, like the United Kingdom, has to import most of the food that it eats. This increase in imported commodities, plus the decline by 28 per cent in the international price of copper, which represented 80 per cent of the Chilean foreign exchange earnings, created a rapid shortage of foreign exchange and a rapid worsening in Chile's balance of payments.

Compounding this situation, there was the "invisible" economic blockade, which started immediately after the UP government took office. As Steenland (39, p. 10) points out, to fully understand the meaning of this economic blockade, you have to realize that in Chile, a country with a gross national product of about $10 billion, a government budget of about $700 million and exports of about $1 billion, United States investments also amounted to a sizable $1 billion, controlling 20 per cent of the Chilean industry, with participation in another 7 per cent. Steenland (39, p. 14) continues:

> In the dominant industries, foreign interests controlled 30.4 percent and participated in another 13.2 percent . . . And aside from outright control through ownership, Chilean industry used largely U.S. machinery and was dependent on the U.S. for technology. This dependency was greatest where the industries were most modern, and in industries which were growing rapidly—rubber, electric machines, refinement of metals, and lumber. In addition to U.S. control through technology and ownership, the U.S. government also exercised great indirect economic power through international finance institutions.

Not surprisingly, then, when the Allende government nationalized the U.S.-dominated mining industry, the United States pressured the international lending institutions to deny new credits to the Chilean economy, with the result that the total loans and credits fell in just one year—1971—from $525 million to just over $30 million. (For an excellent and detailed account of the economic blockade, see reference 47.) The Santiago correspondent of the Washington *Post* (48, p. 1, 14), writing just

[10]One of the goods whose consumption increased most as a result of the growth in purchasing power of the working class and peasantry was beef. Under the Alessandri administration (1958–1964) a worker had to labor five hours, 35 minutes to buy a kilo of stewing beef; under Frei, four hours, 53 minutes; but under the UP, a worker had to labor only two hours to buy the same amount (46).

after the coup described how the economic blockade helped to cripple the Allende administration:

> Since 1970, the Allende government has been the target of economic policies that have squeezed the fragile Chilean economy to the choking point. These policies were conceived in an atmosphere of economic strife between the Allende government and a group of large U.S. corporations whose Chilean holdings were nationalized under the terms of Allende's socialist platform. The instruments for carrying out the sustained program of economic pressure against Allende were the U.S. foreign aid program, the Inter American Development Bank, the U.S. Export Import Bank, the World Bank and also private U.S. banking institutions . . . [one example of this blockade is that] one of the first actions under the new policy was the denial by the Export Import Bank of a request for $21 million in credit to finance purchase of three Boeing passenger jets by the Chilean government airline, LAN-Chile. The credit position of the airline, according to a U.S. official familiar with the negotiations, was an excellent one.[11]

These credits were needed to buy not only foodstuffs, but also machinery, equipment, etc., and also to pay off the $3 billion foreign debt that the Frei government had left the nation, which made Chile the second most indebted country per capita in the world, after Israel (39, p. 14). The lumpenbourgeoisie, dependent on foreign capital, joined the external boycott with an internal one together with explicitly political strikes, increasingly aimed at causing the fall of the UP government or triggering a military coup. One part of this boycott was the truck owners' strike that paralyzed the system of transport and hindered food distribution, thus compounding existing scarcities (39, p. 16).

It was thus the greatly increased demand for basic goods and services plus the politically motivated shortages, the result of both the international blockade and the lumpenbourgeoisie boycott, that determined the need to ration those basic goods. And not unlike rationing in other countries, the ones more opposed to that rationing were the upper rather than the lower classes. For the lower classes, the "free market" supported by the wealthy was in itself a form of rationing where the criteria for the distribution of food was based on the consumer power of the rich. Thus, the lower classes were far more sympathetic to formal rationing, where the criteria for the distribution of resources were defined by a government that was, at least in theory, sympathetic to their needs. And according to an opinion poll published in the weekly paper *Ercilla* (49), which was of anti-UP sympathies, the success of the Allende government distribution

---

[11]As a footnote to this report, incidentally, I might add that the credit to buy these Boeing jets was granted just two weeks *after* the coup.

policies was shown by the fact that while 75 per cent of those lower-class householders polled said that essential goods had become easier to obtain, 77 per cent of middle-class and 93 per cent of high-income households were finding them less accessible. The medical profession, very much a part of these latter classes, was among those who were finding the essential goods less accessible.

As a Chilean folk song says,

> sharing the riches, my son, is for some to have less and for others to have more.

And the period 1970–1973 in Chile saw an attempt to redefine this idea of sharing. Not surprisingly, the medical profession and the classes it belonged to, the lumpenbourgeoisie and the middle classes, did not want to have their class and professional privileges redefined. Nor were they willing to tolerate the integration of health services into one system that would have determined the sharing of their resources with the majority of Chileans.

The Fall of the Allende Administration

As I have explained, it was in the delay in bringing about the integration of the two-class medicine into one health system that the UP government showed its greatest hesitancy in the health sector, although this hesitancy seems to have been a "trademark" of the Allende administration in other areas as well. Actually, as Sweezy (41) has noted, the political strategy of the UP government seems to have been to increase its popular support while trying to avoid or postpone the confrontation with the lumpenbourgeoisie and middle classes. This strategy seemed a valid one in the first year of the administration, when the parties forming the UP coalition, which had polled 36.3 per cent of the vote in the presidential election, just five months later, in April 1971, increased their share of the vote to 51.0 per cent in a municipal election run in terms of support or opposition to the UP government (39, p. 10).

The weakness of this strategy, however, was that it meant postponement not only of the integration of the health services, but also of promised policies in other sectors, and this gave the medical profession and other groups and classes the time to organize their opposition, first, during the year 1972, legally, and later, in 1973, illegally. Indeed, as Sweezy (41) and Petras (42) have indicated, the UP seemed to have underestimated the power of the response of the national bourgeoisie and its international counterparts. A summary list of events shows this. (For a detailed list of events during the Allende administration, see references 13, 38, 39, 40, and 47.)

In October 1972, the truck owners staged their first strike against the government, in theory to delay any attempt by the administration to nationalize transport, but in practice to force the resignation of the government. The medical profession, following a call by the Chilean Medical Association, followed with a strike that was in theory to protest the lack of availability of equipment in the health sector, but, again, in practice, it was meant to force the Allende government to resign. In fact, organized medicine did call for the resignation of Allende at this time. A passing but interesting note here is that the public health physicians, with a great number of faculty and students from the School of Public Health, as well as the majority of the trade unions of health workers, came to the support of the government. Their rallying call, which was to become a slogan later on, was the very non-sectarian one of "this government is shit, but it is our government." The strike did not succeed.

The next great moment of difficulty for Allende's government was in July 1973, when the second strike of the truck owners took place with the explicit aim of either causing the fall of Allende or stimulating a military coup. The medical profession joined in with renewed requests for Allende's resignation. And, in an almost unanimous resolution, the Chilean Medical Association decided to expel President Allende from its membership. Dr. Allende, I might mention here, had been one of the first officers of the association when it was founded.

Meanwhile, from the end of 1972, as was recently announced by the present military leaders and reported by the New York *Times* (1), the truck owners, the professionals (including the Chilean Medical Association), the Chilean Chamber of Commerce, and other groups representative of the economic interests, national and international, had been planning, together with the military leaders, the final military coup of September 11, 1973, which achieved what they had been asking for, the fall of the Unidad Popular government.[12] The Chilean Medical Associa-

[12]It has been said, particularly by conservative voices, that the military coup was a necessary response to the "lawlessness of the masses," which seems to be their code name for the mass mobilization of the lower classes. This argument deliberately ignores the documented fact, recognized even by the junta itself, that the military started planning the coup as early as six months after Allende's administration took office and one year before the spontaneous mobilization of the working class took place. Moreover, the first mass mobilization occurred, as indicated in the text, after, not before, the first (unsuccessful) coup took place. In that respect, the historical sequence shows that the mobilization was a response by the working class to the military and strike threats from the lumpenbourgeoisie and the armed forces, not vice versa.

tion was the first professional association to send a telegram of support to the junta, applauding its "patriotism."

It seems, then, that the fear and hesitancy of the Allende government also brought about its end. The leadership's belief that time and, thus, evolution were on their side apparently proved, ultimately, to be a self-defeating strategy.[13] The dramatic successes of the first year and the great popularity of the government during that year were not used to advantage, to implement in each sector of the economy such policies as the integration of the health services that, by strengthening UP aims and policies, would have weakened its opponents.

The Response of the Reaction[14]

Not surprisingly, the military junta, the voice of those interests which were curtailed during the Allende administration, including those of the medical profession, has undone most of the advances that the working class and peasantry achieved during the period 1970–1973. This has taken place both outside as well as inside the health sector. Let me list some of the most important changes brought about by the junta.

First, the project of integrating the two-class medicine has been abandoned, with a declared commitment by the junta to leave the fee-for-service system of payment in SERMENA untouched. There has even been talk within the military circles of changing the system of payment to physicians within the National Health Service from salary to fee-for-service (50). A colonel has been appointed Minister of Health and the treasurer of the Chilean Medical Association has been appointed Director General of the National Health Service.

In other sectors of the economy, the junta has returned to the initial owners, to the private sector, most of the industries nationalized during the UP administration (51) and said that it would pay for the remaining ones on generous terms (52). According to an interview with General Pinochet, the head of the junta, published in *La Prensa* (53), the leadership wants to open negotiations with the U.S. ex-owners of the nationalized copper mines on terms favorable to the U.S. companies,

[13]The main architect of this evolutionary strategy within the coalition of the Unidad Popular parties was the Communist Party.

[14]Information published in this section relies very heavily on the dispatches from the correspondents in Chile of the *New York Times, Washington Post,* and *Le Monde,* as well as information from Chilean and other witnesses who were part of these events. Additional information is from Sweezy (41); Petras (42); Scientists and Engineers for Social and Political Action (13); North American Congress on Latin America (40 and 47).

since "it is not ethical that we Chileans take over what does not belong to us." Also, an economic policy has been established aimed at encouraging foreign investments on terms very favorable and generous to foreign capital. Furthermore, a policy has been instituted that is deliberately aimed at welcoming foreign investments, mimicking the "brotherly regime of Brazil" (54, p. 12). And just one month after the coup, the World Bank (which had denied loans to Chile for three years), together with the Inter American Bank, loaned $260 million to the new government. As the president of the Chilean Bank, General Eduardo Cano, has said, "the World Bank and international financial circles were well disposed to the new military government in Chile" (55, p. A 32).

Further proof of this good will is that the Latin American Development Bank, which turned down every request made by the Allende government, awarded a development loan to the junta that is almost five times the size of all loans received during the Allende administration (2).[15] One month after the coup, the Nixon administration in the United States approved a $24 million credit to the junta, for the purchase of 120,000 tons of wheat. This credit, as Senator Kennedy indicated on the floor of the U.S. Senate (57, p. A 11),

> was eight times the total commodity offered to Chile in the past three years when a democratically elected government was in power.

Second, the coup, which was a bonanza for the Chilean lumpenbourgeoisie and middle classes and their international counterparts, has meant belt-tightening for the working class and peasantry in the health sector and other sectors of the nation.

In the health sector, institutional democracy was automatically discontinued a week after the coup. And the Minister of Public Health declared that in matters of policy, the military would rely "very heavily on the good judgment and patriotic commitment of the Chilean Medical Association" (58). At the same time, the Chilean Medical Association sent a delegation abroad to several foreign countries, including Uruguay, Brazil, and the United States, to strengthen a scientific exchange with their professional colleagues and equivalent organizations in those countries. The Chilean Medical Association also reassured the military junta of its complete support (59).

Outside the health sector, the junta discontinued the workers' control

---

[15]Also, according to *U.S. News and World Report* (56), U.S. bankers have decided to provide short-term loans to private and government banks totaling $39 million, to aid the Chilean economy.

of the management of the factories, returning them to the previous managers and, at the same time, banned trade unions, incarcerating the national leaders of the trade unions, including those of the health worker unions. In addition, all political party activities were forbidden, and all working-class-based parties were outlawed. Only those the junta defines as "patriots" are entitled to any form of civil rights. The narrowness of its definition may be best reflected by the declaration of General Pinochet accusing "the U.S. Senate of being under the influence of international communism" (60).

Third, the junta changed the priorities in the health services. The amount of resources available to the health centers was reduced and the amount available to the hospitals increased. The number of hours that physicians have to spend in health centers was halved, and the hours the centers are open to the public were shortened to the 8:00 A.M. to 4:00 P.M. schedule of pre-Allende times. Moreover, the milk distribution program was discontinued.

Outside the health sector, price controls were discontinued and the goods desired by the upper and middle classes are now plentiful in the stores. The working class and peasantry, meanwhile, as reported by the New York *Times* (61, p. 10) are going through very tough times of tight budgeting.

Fourth, all opposition was outlawed and persecuted, and in the health sector a campaign of repression was begun against those physicians and health workers who did not join the physicians' strike against Allende's government, who were considered sympathetic to Allende, and whose names were provided to the police authorities by the Chilean Medical Association (62). Also, a campaign of repression was started against the public health movement, which, by and large, supported the Allende administration. The budget of Chile's only school of public health, which is situated in Santiago and is the most prestigious school of its kind in Latin America, was slashed by three-quarters, and 82 faculty members out of a total of 110 were fired and some imprisoned (63). As the Chilean Ministry of Public Health (64) says, "Very many public health workers were misguided and their activities were subversive of the traditional medical values." In Chile, also, the medical schools and all other university centers have been placed under military control. All presidents and deans of academic institutions are now military men. As Dr. E. Boeninger, the last president of the University of Chile, said, "The Chilean University is in the hands of the military" (65).

Known results of this repression in the health field are that, in the first six months following the coup, 21 physicians were shot, 85 imprisoned, and countless others dismissed (66).

Outside the health sector, the junta has instituted a campaign of repression that has been defined by Amnesty International as the most brutal that that association has ever surveyed, more brutal even than the repression in Brazil in 1965, Greece in 1968, and Uruguay in 1972 (67). Today, ten months after the coup, the state of siege continues (68).

Epilogue

It may be too soon to make a post mortem of the performance of the Allende administration in the health sector. But still, enough knowledge of those years has been accumulated to entitle us to draw some conclusions. And perhaps one important interpretation of these events is that Chile seems to show, once again, what Brazil, the Dominican Republic, Uruguay, Paraguay, Bolivia, and many, many other Latin American countries have shown before—that there is a rigidity in the economic, political, and social structures of most Latin American countries that makes change almost an impossibility, however slow or gradual that change may be. The lumpenbourgeoisie and their foreign counterparts offer extremely strong opposition to any movement that might imply the curtailment of their benefits, however slow or minimal this curtailment may be. They perceive that any concession has a momentum of its own and that it might escalate, according to the sadly famous "domino theory," to the final destruction of their privileges.

The reaction of these groups to the UP government in Chile is an example of this. Actually, in spite of the alarm that the Unidad Popular administration created in many U.S. corridors of power, Allende's government was not a "radical" one. As the pro-UP economist Alberto Martinez indicated, even if all the programs for nationalization that the UP government called for had been implemented, it would have meant state control of only 25 per cent of industrial production outside of the mining sector, which is less than the control of that production by U.S. interests, estimated to be close to 30 per cent (39, p. 12). In fact, Allende (69, p. C 1) himself argued:

> I want to insist that Chile is not a socialist country. This is a capitalist country and my government is not a socialist government. This is a popular, democratic, national revolutionary government—anti-imperialist.

Indeed, he emphasized that the UP was an "anti-imperialist and antimonopolistic government, more than a socialist one" (70, p. 85). And, again, he held that it was "not a socialist government, rather, there is a government that is going to open the path, to blaze the path for socialism" (71).

The major economic decisions taken by Allende were the nationalization of the copper industry and the takeover of the control of banking and most of the foreign commerce, measures that were more of an antioligarchical and nationalist than of a socialist nature. Concerning his interior policies, a UP economist (44, p. 17) has explained that Allende's economic policy was similar to what we in the United States

> would call the New Deal type . . . [since] it combines a policy of large-scale public works (especially housing and related services) with fiscal and monetary measures designed to stimulate popular purchasing power . . . [and with] strict price controls [which] would keep these gains from being dissipated as has regularly been the case in the past, through inflation.

Not surprisingly, Allende has been called the Léon Blum of Chile. And, actually, his reforms could hardly be accused of being an intrinsic threat to the capitalist system. In spite of this, however, the national and international interests perceived his programs as being the beginning of the end for them. And the opposition to those UP economic policies was formidable, showing how, inside the parameters of underdevelopment and within the present structures, the possibilities for change, however limited, are very small indeed. It does seem as if Allende underestimated this opposition. The gradualism and the faith of the leadership of the UP in the "uniqueness" of the Chilean phenomenon (considered by some to be unhistorical), together with its postponement of outright decisions that would have weakened its opponents, apparently allowed time for the massive opposition of the national and international interests to organize.[16] The postponement of the integration of health services is a fitting case in point.

In that respect, Allende's delays may have also caused his downfall. And, contrary to prevalent belief in some sectors of the U.S. press, Allende's downfall may have been brought about not so much because he went too fast, but because he went too slowly. Indeed, as Oskar Lange (73) said almost forty years ago, if

> a socialist government . . . declares that the textile industry is going to be

[16]As an ITT memorandum indicated, "a realistic hope among those who want to block Allende is that a swiftly deteriorating economy . . . will touch off a wave of violence, resulting in a military coup" (72, p. A 2).

socialized after five years, we can be quite certain that the textile industry will be ruined before it will be socialized . . . [during those five years] no government supervision or administrative measures can cope effectively with the passive resistance and sabotage of the owners and managers.

It is my belief that this observation applied to the health sector as well as to other areas. Indeed, in the health sector, many proposals for national health insurance schemes and/or national health services have been frustrated because of delays in their implementation and because of final compromises with the medical profession and with other interest groups in the health sector. Actually, the Chilean experience only reflects previous experience in other countries, be they socialist or capitalist: when a political party or group is committed to a national health program intended to benefit the citizenry and to curtail the privileges of the providers, its chances of implementation are inversely related to the length of time required for implementation. We can see that, in Chile, the longer the delay, the more time there was for the interest groups to organize and achieve compromises that diluted and subtracted from the program. And these compromises, I might add, can only benefit the providers, not the consumers, the majority of the citizenry.

There are certain conclusions, then, that we can derive from the events in Chile. One is that the present political structures in most of Latin America (and, I would add, in most of the underdeveloped world) hinder, rather than foster, any opportunity to bring about a change that would benefit not just the few, but the many. The national and international economic elites control those political structures to maintain outdated and grossly unjust political, social, and economic privileges in opposition to the popular demands of the majority of the population. A second conclusion would be that gradualism by those parties and groups in underdeveloped countries that are committed to change weakens the possibilities for change in the health sector and in other areas. The Chilean workers and peasants, the real heroes of the tragedy that was played out in Chile, clearly understood this when they kept urging the Allende government to proceed with reform at a faster pace. And when, after the first, unsuccessful, military coup, Chilean society began increasingly to polarize, the working class and peasantry, in their working places, their factories, their hospitals and health centers, and in their communities, began to mobilize and to prepare themselves for the coming second coup. In a battle against time, they have lost for the time being, and the privileged classes and their military brute force have won. As Neruda (74, p. 111) said almost forty years ago, on the day that another military coup took place, in Spain, hope lived in the hearts of the people

Till one morning everything blazed:
one morning bonfires
sprang out of earth
and devoured all the living;
since then, only fire;
since then, the blood and the gunpowder,
ever since then.

Bandits in airplanes
and marauders with seal rings and duchesses
black friars and brigands signed with the cross, coming
out of the clouds to a slaughter of innocents.

References

1. Kandell, J., Military junta in Chile prohibits Marxist parties, *New York Times,* September 22, 1973, p. 1; Chilean officers tell how they began to plan the takeover last November, *New York Times,* September 27, 1973, p. 3; Ousted bosses back at Chile's plants, *New York Times,* September 25, 1973, p. 3.; Chile offers to reopen talks on copper, *New York Times,* September 29, 1973, p. 3.

2. Birns, L.R. Chile in the *Wall Street Journal. Nation* 217: 581–587, 1973.

3. Support of the professional organizations for the revolutionary government. *El Mercurio,* September 18, 1973. (In Spanish)

4. The Chilean coup. *Le Monde Diplomatique,* October 13–17, 1973. (In French)

5. Navarro, V. The underdevelopment of health or the health of underdevelopment: an analysis of the distribution of human health resources in Latin America. *Politics and Society* 4(2):267–293, 1974. (Also included on pp. 3–32 of this volume.)

6. Johnson, D.L., editor. *The Chilean Road to Socialism.* Anchor Press, New York, 1973.

7. Frank, A.G. *Lumpenbourgeoisie: Lumpendevelopment. Dependence, Class, and Politics in Latin America.* Monthly Review Press, New York and London, 1972.

8. Petras, J. *Politics and Social Structure in Latin America.* Monthly Review Press, New York and London, 1970.

9. Frank, A.G. *Capitalism and Underdevelopment in Latin America: Historical Studies of Chile and Brazil.* Monthly Review Press, New York and London, 1969.

10. Chilean Ministry of Public Health. *Human Resources in the Health Sector in Chile.* National Health Service Press, Santiago, 1970. (In Spanish)

11. Gaete, J. and Castanon, R. *The Development of the Medical Care Institutions in Chile During This Century.* University of Chile, Santiago. (In Spanish)

12. Diaz, S. Family health expenditures. *Cuadernos Medico-Sociales* VII(4):21–26, 1966. (In Spanish)

13. Scientists and Engineers for Social and Political Action. Chile. *Bulletin of the Scientists and Engineers for Social and Political Action* 5(6), 1973.

14. Chilean Ministry of Public Health. *The National Health Service.* Subdepartment of Health Education, Santiago, 1950. (In Spanish)

15. Sigerist, H.E. *Landmarks in the History of Hygiene.* Oxford University Press, London, 1956.

16. Terris, M. Crisis and change in America's health system. *American Journal of Public Health* 65:313–318, 1973.

17. Laval, E. The biography of Don Alejandro del Rio. *Journal of Social Welfare* XIII, 1944. (In Spanish)

18. Laval, E. and Garcia, R. Synthesis of the historical development of public health in Chile. *Journal of the National Health Service* 1, 1956. (In Spanish)

19. Hall, T.L. and Diaz, S. Social security and health care patterns in Chile. *International Journal of Health Services* 1 (4):362–377, 1971.

20. Requena, M. Program of ambulatory medical care in the National Health Service, Report of the Director-General of Health. Ministry of Public Health, Santiago, 1971.

21. Sepulveda, P.S. Perspectives for a revolutionary change in Chilean medical care. University of Chile, Santiago, 1973. (In Spanish)

22. Cockcroft, J., Frank, A.G. and Johnston, D.L. *Dependence and Underdevelopment: Latin America's Political Economy.* Doubleday, New York, 1972.

23. de Ahumada, J. *Health Planning for Latin America.* Pan American Health Organization, Washington, D.C., 1968.

24. Navarro, V. and Ruderman, A.P., editors. Health and socioeconomic development. Special issue of *International Journal of Health Services* 1 (3), 1971.

25. Feinberg, R.E. *The Triumph of Allende: Chile's Legal Revolution.* Mentor Books, New York, 1972.

26. Chilean Ministry of Public Health. *Levels of Medical Care.* Fifth Zone of the National Health Service. Santiago, 1972. (In Spanish)

27. Sheps, C. The influence of consumer sponsorship on medical services. *Milbank Memorial Fund Quarterly* 50(4):41–69, 1972.

28. Weaver, N.D.W. Community participation in the welfare state and hospitals. *The Hospital* 67:347–351, 1971.

29. Great Britain, Ministry of Health. *National Health Service Reorganization: England.* Her Majesty's Stationery Office (Command 5055), London, 1972.

30. Chilean Trade Unions of Health Workers. *Political Organization of the Community, Popular Power and Democratization of Health.* First Congress of the Trade Unions of Health Workers, Santiago, 1971. (In Spanish)

31. Germara, C. The state and the marginal masses in Chile. *Bolletin ELAS* 4(6), 1970. (In Spanish)

32. Unidad Popular Party. *Political Platform of the Unidad Popular Party.* Unidad Popular Press, Santiago, 1970. (In Spanish)

33. Albala, C. and Santander, P. *Preliminary Study of the Process of Democratization in the National Health Service.* University of Chile, Santiago, 1972. (In Spanish)

34. Miliband, R. *The State in Capitalist Society.* Weidenfeld and Nicolson, London, 1969.

35. Crossman, R. *Inside View: Three Lectures on Prime Ministerial Government.* Jonathan Cape, London, 1972.

36. Myrdal, G. *Beyond the Welfare State.* Yale University Press, New Haven, 1960.

37. Robinson, J. *The Cultural Revolution in China.* Penguin Books, Baltimore, 1969.

38. Zimbalist, A. and Stallings, B. Showdown in Chile. *Monthly Review* 25(5):1–24, 1973.

39. Steenland, K. Two years of "Popular Unity" in Chile: a balance sheet. *New Left Review* 78: 3–25, 1973.

40. North American Congress on Latin America. Chile: the story behind the coup. Issue of *Latin America and Empire Report* VII (8), 1973.

41. Sweezy, P.M. Chile: the question of power. *Monthly Review* 25 (7):1–11, 1973.

42. Petras, J. Chile after Allende: a tale of two coups. *Monthly Review* 25(7):12–20, 1973.

43. Rojas, R. The Chilean armed forces: the role of the military in the Popular Unity government. In Johnson, D.L., editor. *The Chilean Road to Socialism.* Anchor Press, New York, 1973.

44. Monthly Review Editors. Peaceful transition to socialism? *Monthly Review* 22(8):1–18, 1971.

45. Rosenstein-Rodan, P.N. Allende's big failing: incompetence. *New York Times,* June 16, 1974.

46. North American Congress on Latin America. *New Chile.* NACLA, Berkeley and New York, 1972.

47. North American Congress on Latin America. Chile facing the blockade. Issue of *Latin America and Empire Report* VII (1), 1973.

48. U. S. puts credit squeeze on Allende government. *Washington Post,* September 24, 1973.

49. *Ercilla.* September 13–19, 1973: 10 (In Spanish)

50. Chilean Ministry of Public Health. *Bulletin No. 35.* Government Printing Office, Santiago, 1973. (In Spanish)

51. Chileans draft recovery plan. *Washington Post,* September 24, 1973.

52. Kandell, J. Chile offers to reopen talks on copper. *New York Times,* September 29, 1973.

53. Interview with General Pinochet. *LaPrensa,* October 22, 1973. (In Spanish)

54. *Washington Post,* November 19, 1973.

55. Chile claims favor of West's bankers. *Washington Post,* October 8, 1973.

56. Links with Chile revive. *U.S. News and World Report,* December 3, 1973. p. 85.

57. Chile gets U.S. loan for wheat. *Washington Post,* October 6, 1973.

58. Chilean Ministry of Public Health. *Bulletin No. 38.* Government Printing Office, Santiago, 1973 (In Spanish)

59. Starting anew in curative medicine. *El Mercurio,* November 9, 1973. (In Spanish)

60. General Pinochet said that the U.S. Senate is under the influence of Communism. *La Prensa,* October 22, 1973. (In Spanish)

61. Kandell, J. Chile four months later. *New York Times,* January 28, 1974.

62. Argus, A. Medicine and politics in Chile. *World Medicine,* April 10, 1974.

63. Ad Hoc Committee to Save Chilean Health Workers, American Public Health Association. Unpublished Letter, December, 1973.

64. Chilean Ministry of Public Health. *Bulletin No. 16.* Government Printing Office, Santiago, 1973. (In Spanish)

65. Military delegates in universities. *El Mercurio,* September 29, 1973. (In Spanish)

66. An appeal from Chilean medical doctors in exile. Letter sent from Lima, Peru, March, 1974.

67. Terror in Chile. *New York Review of Books* XXI:38–44. May 30, 1974.

68. Gott, R. Chile keeps state of siege. *Manchester Guardian Weekly* 110, June 29, 1974, p. 7.

69. Chile's Allende: a prophetic interview. *Washington Post,* September 28, 1973.

70. Debray, R. *The Chilean Revolution: Conversations with Allende.* Vintage Books, New York, 1971.

71. Allende, S. Interview on "Meet the Press," October 13, 1971.

72. *Washington Post,* September 16, 1973.

73. Lange, O. On the economic theory of socialism. *Monthly Review* 22(8): 38–44, 1971.

74. Neruda, P. A few things explained. In *The Selected Poems of Pablo Neruda,* translated by B. Belitt. Grove Press, New York, 1963.

Health and Medicine in the Rural United States: Its Political and Economic Determinants

To the coal miners of Appalachia and
to the migrant workers of Florida,
whose underdevelopment of health
shares the same causation.

The Underdevelopment of Health in Rural America

In our daily debates on problems and possible solutions for this United States of ours, we tend to overlook that, however urban our society may be, 26 per cent of our population, or not less than 55 million Americans, continue to live in the rural U.S. In this paper, I will examine very briefly, first, the health conditions of rural America, with main emphasis on the rural poor; second, the reasons, as I perceive them, for those conditions; and third, some suggestions for improving them.

Let me begin, then, with a very brief sketch of the health conditions of rural America, starting with an analysis of infant mortality, one fairly good indicator of such conditions.

Figure 1 shows the infant mortality rate for the ten highest-income urban states, the ten lowest-income rural states, the three poorest rural states, and the rural counties of West Virginia. And it shows that the infant mortality rate in the poorest rural areas, such as the rural counties of West Virginia, is double that in the highest-income urban states. In other words, the probability of an infant dying during his first year of life is twice as great in the poorest rural areas than in the wealthiest urban states. Moreover, the gap between the poorest and wealthiest, measured by number of preventable infant deaths, has been increasing rather than declining over the last ten years.

If, instead of looking at the number of deaths among infants, we look at the number of deaths among their mothers (i.e. maternal mortality), the findings are equally striking. Indeed, while women living in rural America make up only 20 per cent of all women of fertile age (mothers and potential mothers), they account for 50 per cent of all maternal deaths in the country. The message of these figures on infant and maternal mortality is quite clear: for both infants and mothers, rural America is a rougher place to live and die than is urban America.

Figure 1

Infant Mortality in 1971

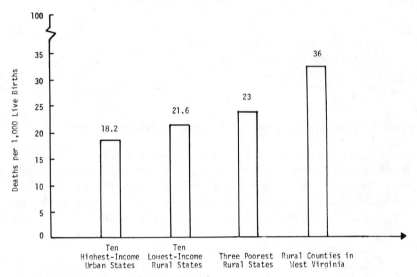

Sources: Estimated from references 1 and 2.

Let me hasten to add that this picture of health, or lack of it, that we have seen for infants and mothers holds true for other age groups as well. Indeed, the proportion of deaths is higher in rural than in urban America for almost all age groups. And, when we look at the causes of that mortality, we find that for those causes associated with poverty (e.g. tuberculosis), the number of deaths in comparable populations is three times as high in the poorest rural areas as it is in the wealthiest urban states (see Figure 2).[1] The same is true, incidentally, for all types of accidents, as also shown in Figure 2.

Let me add a note here that has relevance to the figures on mortality due to accidents. And that is that although the system of collecting information does not allow us to specify how many of those accidents are work-related, still the information that some of us have collected seems, at least tentatively, to show that mortality due to labor accidents is higher in rural America—almost double—than in the urban U.S. (4). And, when we include both rural and urban deaths due to accidents that have

[1]The figures presented in this overview of mortality conditions in rural America were compiled from references 1, 2 and 3.

Figure 2

Rates of Mortality Due to Tuberculosis and Accidents
per 100,000 Population, 1969

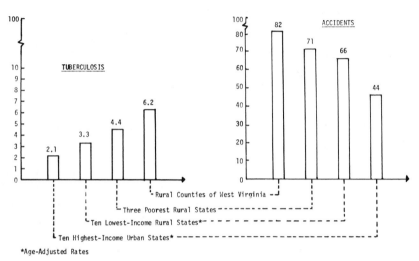

*Age-Adjusted Rates

Sources: Estimated from references 1 and 2.

occurred at the workplace, our record is quite poor compared with that of
other industrialized countries, whether capitalist or socialist (5).

If, instead of mortality, we look at the morbidity picture, i.e. the
prevalence and type of disease in rural America, we find that one of the
most embarrassing—and, I would add, scandalous—health problems in
rural poor America is undernutrition and even hunger. For those who
may find these adjectives too strong, allow me to mention that, as one
reflection of the priorities and irrational way that resources are
distributed in the U.S. economic system, $2.5 billion are annually spent
on pet food (6, p. 58), while "26 million Americans cannot afford to
purchase an adequate diet, and over 11.2 million of them receive no help
whatever from any federal food program" (7, p. 9). And the majority of
these Americans live in rural America. Actually, a recent nationwide
nutritional survey carried out by the U.S. Department of Agriculture
showed that about 23 per cent of all rural householders had diets that
were poor, i.e. diets that supplied less than two-thirds of the recommended
allowances for one or more nutrients (8). That percentage is far higher

and the nutritional deficiencies—including hunger—even larger, in the poor rural states (7). The recognition of this fact led to the introductory statement to the report of the 1969 White House Conference on Food, Nutrition and Health: "Hunger exists on a disgraceful scale in the United States" (9). As that great woman and labor leader, Mother Jones, said, "Reality speaks for itself. And reality is sometimes quite strong!"

This, then, is the picture of health, or, more precisely defined, lack of health, of significant portions of rural America. And although there are some joys, day to day life in today's rural America is more often one of much misery, death and disease.

The Distribution of Health Resources in Rural America: Scarcity and Maldistribution

We find the same situation in the distribution of resources in the health sector that we find outside it, i.e. the greater the need for resources, the lower their availability. As the Presidential Commission on Rural Poverty, set up in 1967 by President Johnson, reported, "Nowhere in the United States is the need for health services so acute, and nowhere is it so inadequate [and unavailable as in rural America]." This statement, incidentally, is almost identical to that concluding the report of President Theodore Roosevelt's Commission on Country Life, published in 1910. "Theoretically," that report noted, "the farm should be the most healthful place in which to live . . . but it is a fact that . . . health conditions in many parts of the open country . . . are in urgent need of betterment" (quoted in 3). And both statements apply equally to rural America today, where 26 per cent of the population is being served by only 12 per cent of the nation's doctors and 18 per cent of the nurses (3). And, not surprisingly, that relative lack of health resources is most highly concentrated among the rural poor. As one example, in 1965, there were sixty communities in West Virginia with fewer than 10,000 inhabitants having no physician whatsoever (2). And the picture is not much better in preventive services. For example, according to a recent survey by the Virginia Department of Health, 52 per cent of the children under two years of age in that state have not received any form of immunization against polio, tetanus, measles, rubella, diphtheria, whooping cough, and other diseases (10).

But bad as the availability of resources (both curative and preventive) in the medical care sector may be, the situation is even worse with respect to environmental health resources that, in my opinion, are more important in optimizing the level of health of the population than is medical care. And here again, at the risk of sounding too strong, let me stress that some of the conditions present in rural America are quite similar to those found in underdeveloped countries. For example, in 1968, West Virginia's own Health Task Force identified 60 per cent of all homes in that state as having a system of solid waste disposal hazardous to the health of the public, and 25 per cent of all homes as having inadequate water and sewage systems (2). Those figures present an uncomfortable reality and one which most of the media, in their age and style of celebration, choose to avoid, as though not to shatter the pleasant illusion of the American dream.[2]

Causes of the Underdevelopment of Health in Rural America

Having described, however briefly, the poor health conditions of rural America, let me now address the question of why those conditions exist. And the first thing we have to realize is that in order to understand poverty in rural America, we have to look first at the production and distribution of wealth in urban America. Indeed, one of the basic facts that we have to recognize in order to explain the situation and conditions in rural poor America is that those areas are not poor because they do not have resources. Quite to the contrary, and reflecting the sad paradox of our economic system, those poor areas are very wealthy indeed, supplying many of the country's raw materials and agricultural products. Indeed, the economic reality is that most of our country's industrial wealth is based on products coming from rural America, including rural poor America.

Let me illustrate this apparent paradox with two examples. The first one is Appalachia. People living and working in Appalachia are very poor. Their infant mortality is more than 50 per cent above the national average, and the mortality due to accidents at the workplace among coal miners—an important sector of the labor force in that region—is the highest in the country, and, incidentally, higher than in most European countries, both Western and Eastern.[3] While not given to hyperboles, I can find no better expression to define the very poor safety conditions in coal mining than "appalling." Actually,

[2]For an interesting discussion of the upper class and urban biases of most of our media, see reference 11.

[3]For detailed information on health conditions in Appalachia, see references 12, 13 and 14.

in the 100 years that partial records of fatal mine accidents have been kept (the early figures are incomplete) more than 120,000 men have died violently in coal mines, an average of 100 every month for a century (quoted in reference 15).

Even today, on the average, one miner is killed every other day in U.S. coal mines, and a very large percentage of those deaths take place in Appalachia (16).

But Appalachia, with its many poor and sick people, and with many preventable deaths, is not poor. Seventy per cent of the coal used most of Eastern industry comes from Appalachia, and the coal indus based to a large degree on coal coming from Appalachia—is one most profitable industries in the country. Moreover, the coal indus Appalachia is dominated by a few large firms that are owne corporations outside the region. In fact,

> coal is more and more under the control of international petroleum providing a direct link between Appalachia and many Third World countries. Rick Diehl's study of the international energy elite shows that Consolidation Coal, the region's largest producer, is owned by Continental Oil Company; that Island Creek Coal Company, which is second in output, is owned by the California-based Occidental Petroleum Corporation; and the third largest producer in the region, Eastern Associated, is a wholly-owned subsidiary of a Boston holding company called Eastern Gas and Fuel Associates. About 10 percent of Appalachia coal output comes from so-called "captive" mines owned by US Steel, Bethlehem Steel and other national steel firms (17).

And it is important to note that those corporations, which are among the main components of the corporate structure in this country, take away from Appalachia far more than they invest in it.[4] For example, in 1967, the net outflow of capital that left Appalachia, i.e. the difference between the capital coming into and leaving Appalachia via those corporations was $54 million (17). We find then, in Appalachia, the same situation that André Gunder Frank (20), Pierre Jallé (21) and others have found in underdeveloped countries: corporate capital absorbs like a sponge the resources and wealth that exist in those countries, taking away more, far more, than is given back.[5] Similarly, corporate capital absorbs the wealth from our rural poor areas. This situation has been defined by

[4]For excellent information on the economic conditions of Appalachia, see the various issues of *People's Appalachia* (such as references 14 and 17), as well as references 18 and 19.
[5]For a more detailed discussion of this point, see reference 23.

Barry Commoner as one of colonization, i.e. "the giant industrial corporations have [indeed] made a colony out of rural America" (quoted in 22). And, as Sara Sanborn recently wrote, within this master-colony relationship, "an economic feast [exists] at which the uninvited guests (the corporations) get the meat and the host (the people of Appalachia) gets the ruined carcass" (15, p. 2).

In summary, since most of American industrial machinery is based on raw materials from Appalachia and other underdeveloped areas, one can postulate that people in Appalachia are poor not because Appalachia has no resources—which it has, and very many at that—but because people in Appalachia have no control whatsoever over those resources.

Indeed, if the Appalachian people could control the resources in their own area, it is highly unlikely that they would be so poor and so unhealthy, or that so little attention would be paid to safety at work in the mines. Moreover, were people in Appalachia able to control the coal mines, it is equally unlikely that the amount of money per miner going to study ways of improving safety in the mines and the occupational health of the miners in Appalachia would be only one-twentieth of that spent in the majority of European countries, as is the case today (14). One can be quite certain that the people in Appalachia would be much more concerned with preventing work-related mortality and sickness among their fathers and sons working in the mines than are the present coal industry leaders. In light of this situation, we can conclude that the main cause for the underdevelopment of health in Appalachia is the absence of power and control that people have over the wealth that they produce.

The second example is migrant workers. Three years ago, and as a result of work that I undertook as a consultant to the State Health Planning Agency of Florida, I had the opportunity to study the health conditions among Floridians (24). And, here again, I found the same paradox: poverty and disease existed precisely in those counties in Florida where most of the wealth in that beautiful agricultural state was produced and among precisely the workers that were farming, collecting and producing that wealth—the migrant and agricultural workers, who produce the agricultural products, primarily citrus, on which the most profitable business in Florida is based, the agrobusiness. Furthermore, as the U.S. Senate Subcommittee on Migratory Labor indicated in an excellent report, the same situation replicates itself in all migrant communities in this country, be they in Florida, Texas, or Southern California, where both the living and working conditions among migrant workers are very poor indeed. Their life expectancy is 49 years, 20 per cent less than that for the average American, and the mortality among their infants is 60 per cent above the national average (25).

Let me add here that the protection of all types of agricultural workers at the working place is practically nil. In 1969, the National Safety Council reported that mining and agriculture were among the most hazardous occupations in terms of deaths and accidents on the job, and among those least protected by legislation. In fact, it was not until 1969 that the Federal black lung benefits were established, breaking a deafening legislative silence on the protection of the coal miners. In agriculture, however, there is not even a national reporting system which would record the extent and effect of long-term exposure to pesticides; nor is there a workers' compensation fund to meet claims for medical and unemployment benefits for agricultural workers, be it migrant workers or cotton pickers, or any other type of agricultural workers (26).

And here again, we find that legislative disregard for the working and health conditions of migrants and agricultural workers is just a symptom of their economic and political poverty—poverty that again is due not to the absence of resources in the areas where they live and work (the agrobusiness is one of the most profitable ones in the country), but to their lack of control over those resources that they greatly contribute to produce. Actually, it is the control of their work and the products of their work by others—the corporate leaders of the agrobusiness, whose primary aim is not the welfare of the population they serve nor of the workers they employ, but the optimization of the always ubiquitous profit—that leads to such striking legislative disregard of those who actually produce those goods. Again, however strong that statement may sound, the reality speaks for itself: many of those profits are based on much death and disease.

These two examples, the poor health among miners and among migrant and agricultural workers, underline my main thesis: their poverty and much of their death and disease is produced not by the absence of resources but by the lack of control over the resources that they produce. Consequently, I postulate that the greatest problem in health, work, and life in rural America, and one that replicates itself in urban America as well, is precisely this lack of control by the majority of the population over the resources and wealth they produce and over the institutions they pay for. This lack of control is clearly perceived by the majority of our U.S. urban and rural populations. The latest Harris poll prepared for the Committee on Government Operations of the U.S. Senate, found a degree of powerlessness, cynicism and alienation among the majority of the U.S. population unprecedented in the history of poll-taking by that association (27).

The Lack of Control by the Majority of the Rural (and Urban) Population over the Health Institutions

This lack of control by the majority of the population over the resources they produce or over the institutions they pay for is also found in the health sector. For example, when we analyze the social class composition of the boards of trustees in the health institutions, be they medical teaching institutions or voluntary hospitals, we find that the corporate and upper-middle classes have the dominant influence, and the lower-middle and working classes—which together represent 80 per cent of the population—are virtually excluded from positions of control.[6] The majority of the U.S. population, then, is practically absent in the "corridors of power" of the health sector, which are heavily dominated by an unrepresentative and unaccountable minority, i.e. the corporate and upper-middle classes (28). Considering that the majority of rural Americans belong, either by work or association, to the occupational categories of farm, services, blue collar, or clerical and sales workers (the main components of the working and lower-middle classes), one can see that this working and lower-middle class underrepresentation goes hand in hand with the underrepresentation of the majority of rural America in the "corridors of power."

Let me underline here that this pattern of class dominance appears also in the executive and legislative branches of both federal and state governments. Indeed, 60 per cent of the cabinet members in our U.S. federal government have been either corporate leaders or business managers; and 60 per cent of our Secretaries of Health have had a similar background (28). A similar picture appears in the legislative branch of the federal government. As Hunt and Sherman point out:

> A total of 102 congressmen held stock or well-paying executive positions in banks or other financial institutions; 81 received regular income from law firms that generally represented big businesses. Sixty-three got their income from stock in the top defense contractors; 45, in the giant (federally regulated) oil and gas industries; 22, in radio and television companies; 11, in commercial airlines; and 9, in railroads (29, p. 284).

[6] For a more detailed discussion of this point, and statistics on the social class composition of the health sector, see reference 28.

There is then a pattern of, if not control, dominant influence by the corporate and upper-middle classes in the main decision-making bodies both within and outside the health sector.

We can ask ourselves at this point what the consequences are of that class control. And there are many. It is not my intention to even list them here. Rather, let me suggest the possible relevance of that dominance in the health sector. And perhaps one of the most apparent ones is the race, sex and class composition of our medical students and, as a result, of our medical profession. From 1960 to 1971, for example, the number of women, who represent 51 per cent of the population, grew from 6 to 12 per cent of the medical student body, and the number of blacks, who represent approximately 12 per cent of the population, increased from 3 to 9 per cent during the same period. While much more needs to be done to break down race and sex discrimination, still, one could say that something is being tried—maybe too little, and maybe too late, but at least people are speaking about it, and steps, however timid, are being taken. There is, however, a far more persistent, consistent, and extensive form of discrimination that no one speaks about—class discrimination, i.e. discrimination against the children of both rural and urban working and lower-middle class families. Indeed, and as Kleinbach (30) has found, the percentage of students coming from families whose income is equal to or less than the median family income—a grouping that includes the poorest half of all U.S. families, and approximately the poorest 50 per cent of the entire U.S. population—has remained constantly underrepresented (12 per cent), not only going back to 1960, but even going further back, to 1920, when following the Flexner report, medical schools as we know them now were established. And although it is very difficult to determine the place of residence of the urban or rural students' families, still we can easily postulate that the percentage of students coming from rural lower-middle and working class families has been constantly underrepresented and may even have declined. Let me add that this inequity is most unfortunate, since, according to a recent study carried out by the West Virginia Medical School, 30 per cent of the students coming from rural West Virginia returned to and practiced in the rural areas, against only 2 per cent of those coming from urban America (31).

In summary, then, we find in the health sector the same situation that we find outside the health sector—the majority of the population does not control either the resources they greatly contribute to produce or the institutions they are increasingly paying for. The corporate and upper middle classes, including the medical profession, have dominant influence and even control in the health sector; the majority—the lower-middle and working classes—have not.

Suggestions for Change

If my presentation of the health problem in rural America is an accurate one, and my interpretation of its causation a valid one, then the health problem of rural America could be defined not only in terms of the classical definitions and categories of mortality and morbidity, but also in terms of the lack of power, control, and dominance of the majority of our population, rural and urban, over the resources they produce or the institutions that they pay for. Actually, it is the latter (the skewed and inequitable distribution of economic, political, and social power) that determines the former (the skewed distribution of mortality and morbidity), and not vice versa.

In that respect, we need to think of preventive medicine and public health not only in terms of improving water and sewage systems, or of improving occupational medicine, or of giving more food to the undernourished, but also, and primarily, in terms of a redistribution of economic and political power and resources in our country that would make possible those strategies and those programs. Actually, if historical experience has any value, it would seem to indicate that all those much-needed measures will not take place, and the present conclusions and recommendations of Presidential Commissions will still be valid fifty years from now unless (a) the pattern of control of our institutions, both outside and within the health sector, changes to make all the "corridors of power" far more responsive, representative, and accountable to the majority of our population than they are today. Indeed, the life and health of rural America will improve only to the degree that rural Americans come to control their own institutions, control that they (and also the majority of urban people) do not have today; and (b) the pattern of control over the wealth in this country changes very profoundly, from control by the few to control by the many. Our concern for optimizing the health of the many requires and demands a commitment to those strategies and policies aimed at changing and diluting the control by the few—an arduous, difficult, hazardous, but stimulating and exciting task.

Consistent with that commitment, I suggest that a criteria for action, both within and outside the health sector, be to support those reforms that facilitate the redistribution of economic and political power from the minority to the majority. Let me illustrate this with an example—the present debate on national health insurance. This debate is limited to the funding and regulation of medical care; not considered is the actual ownership of the different components of the health sector. And the main debate seems to be on the focus of that planning and regulation—on whether that focus should be on the private sector, as most of the proposals are advocating, or on the public sector, as the proposal supported by the majority of the unions is suggesting. Let me add that this debate and its importance is not a minor one. Elsewhere, I have argued the merits of the public sector being responsible for the administration of the funding, planning, and regulation of national health insurance (32). But this shift from private to public does not in itself necessarily guarantee that the distribution of power in the health sector will change. Indeed, public sector intervention could actually serve—as Medicare did—to strengthen rather than weaken the present distribution of economic and political power both within and outside the health sector. In that respect, a major weakness of the union-supported NHI proposal is that it does not even touch on the question of control and ownership of our health institutions. I am referring here to the element of accountability and representativeness of the boards of our institutions and of the planning and regulatory agencies. In other words, there is not a single legislative component in that proposal that would change the class dominance over our institutions discussed earlier in this paper. The upper class and upper-middle class will still continue to control those institutions.

My suggestion, then, is to work for the presentation of alternative proposals that would actually change the pattern of control of our institutions—a change not only from the private to the public sector, but also one that gives control of the institutions to those working in them and those served by them. Such a change would require that members of the executive boards of all our health institutions and agencies of regulation and control be elected by producers of services in those institutions and by the citizenry living in the communities served by them.

Let me underline at this point that I am aware, of course, of the rather limited possibilities of a proposal such as this being accepted by the U.S. Congress at the present moment. Both conservative and liberal authors are likely to argue that (a) the majority of the U.S. population has no desire to control those institutions, and thus, the proposal would fall on unreceptive congressional ears, and (b) even were change of control, as suggested here, to take place, the final outcome in terms of overall priorities in the health sector would not be much different from the situation at present.

The first argument, however, makes the assumption that in our political process, the average citizen makes the final choice among informed, diverse, and well-presented alternatives. But increasing evidence, showing a consistent pattern of class dominance in the agencies of communication as well as in the federal executive and legislative bodies of government, makes that assumption a highly questionable one. In fact, it is highly unlikely that a proposal threatening the corporate and upper-middle class dominance of our institutions would have the same opportunity to be meaningfully presented to our citizenry as do others not representing such a threat. The plurality in our system is selectively defined and limited indeed. These obstacles do not obviate, however, the need for continuing the arduous but necessary task of presenting alternatives to our citizenry, toward the end of democratizing our institutions and our society.

With regard to the second point, i.e. raising skepticism as to the effect that democratization of the institutions would have on priorities in the health sector, my answer is that evidence already accumulated in this and other countries shows that when democratization does occur, not as token participation but as control, the pattern of priorities does indeed change (32, 33). Actually, it is because of the real possibility for change that democratization presents that there is so much resistance and opposition to it.

Last, but not least, let me add that the proposal for democratization of the health sector has to be part and parcel of a larger commitment to the democratization of the whole of our society. And that democratization would require a degree of redistribution of economic wealth and political power far, far more profound and massive than is currently envisioned in the major political forums in our country—thus the need for continuously presenting and exploring alternatives. And part of this exploration is to present the issue of workers' and citizens' control, i.e. industrial and institutional democracy, directly and to the point. As André Gorz has indicated, the problem of lack of democracy in our societies can await neither post-industrial society nor socialism. It should be faced in the present (34). And it should be aimed at questioning the prevalent assumptions and mythologies that sustain the system primarily for the benefit of the few and not the many, questioning that should take

place wherever we may be. Indeed, we should heed the words of that folk
song, popular in the hills of Appalachia,

> With plenty of dirty, slaving work, and very little pay
> Coal miner, won't you wake up, and open your eyes and see
> What the dirty profit-seeking system is doing to you and me.
>
> Oh miner, won't you organize wherever you may be
> And make this a land of freedom for workers like you and me.

References

1. Lerner, M. and Stutz, R.N. Have We Narrowed the Gaps Between the Poor and the Nonpoor? Part II: Mortality. Paper presented at the Annual Meeting of the American Public Health Association, New Orleans, 1974.

2. Nolan, R.L. The Rural Health Crisis, 1971. Testimony before the Subcommittee on Health, U.S. Senate, Washington, D.C., March 31, 1971.

3. Margolis, R.J. Notes on the Health of Rural America. Rural Housing Alliance and Rural America, Inc., Washington, D.C., 1975 (mimeographed).

4. Navarro, V., editor. Health Policy Plans for the State of Maryland. Report of the Multidisciplinary Health Planning Program, Johns Hopkins University, Baltimore, 1974.

5. *Occupational Health and Safety, Volumes I and II.* International Labor Organization, Geneva, 1975.

6. The great American animal farm. *Time,* pp. 58–64, December 23, 1974.

7. Citizens Board of Inquiry into Hunger and Malnutrition in the United States. *Hunger U.S.A. Revisited.* National Council on Hunger and Malnutrition and the Southern Regional Council, Atlanta, 1973.

8. United States Congress. *Nutrition and Human Needs.* U.S. Government Printing Office, Washington, D.C., 1969.

9. White House Conference on Food, Nutrition and Health. *Final Report.* U.S. Government Printing Office, Washington, D.C., 1969.

10. Rosenfeld, M. Many Virginia children not getting shots. *Washington Post,* April 27, 1975.

11. Hunter, M. Editor's parley hears criticism, Newspaper editors are told credibility is non-existent—Reader hatred cited. *New York Times,* April 17, 1975.

12. Nolan, R.L., editor. *Rural and Appalachian Health.* Charles C. Thomas, Illinois, 1973.

13. Conte, R.A. *Poverty, Politics and Health Care: An Appalachian Experience.* Praeger, New York, 1975.

14. Coal mine health and safety. *People's Appalachia* 2 (3):38–39. 1975

15. Sanborn, S. Rich songs, poor people. *New York Times Book Review,* April 27, 1974.

16. Research Unit, United Mine Workers, Washington, D.C. Personal communication to the author.

17. Dix, K. Appalachia: third world pillage. *Peoples' Appalachia* 1 (3), 1970.

18. United Mine Workers of America. *Coal Miners and the Economy.* United Mine Workers Research Report, Washington, D.C., 1975.

19. Ridgeway, J. *The Last Play.* Sutton Press, New York, 1973.

20. Frank, A.G. *Lumpenbourgeoisie: Lumpendevelopment.* Monthly Review Press, New York, 1969.

21. Jallé, P. *The Pillage of the Third World.* Monthly Review Press, New York, 1968.

22. Reed, R. Organization formed to speak for rural areas and small towns. *New York Times,* April 21, 1975.

23. Navarro, V. The underdevelopment of health or the health of underdevelopment: an analysis of the distribution of human health resources in Latin America. *International Journal of Health Services* 4(1): 5–27, 1974. (See also pp. 3–32 of this volume.)

24. *The Florida Planning Study for Improved Delivery of Health Services to the Medically Indigent.* Bureau of Comprehensive Health Planning, Florida State Health Department, 1972, mimeographed report.

25. U.S. Congress. *Hearings on Migratory Labor.* U.S. Government Printing Office, Washington, D.C., 1972.

26. Housing Alliance and Rural America, Inc. *Health Services and Rural America,* Washington, D.C., 1975. Mimeographed report.

27. Harris, J. *Confidence and Concern: A Survey of Public Attitudes.* U.S. Government Printing Office, Washington, D.C., 1973.

28. Navarro, V. Social policy issues: an explanation of the composition, nature and functions of the present health sector of the United States. *Bulletin of the New York Academy of Medicine* 51(1): 199–234, 1975. (See also pp. 135–169 of this volume.)

29. Hunt, E.K. and Sherman, H.J. *Economics: An Introduction to Traditional and Radical Views.* Harper and Row, New York, 1972.

30. Kleinbach, G. *Social Class and Medical Education.* (In process).

31. Enticing practitioners to the rural areas. *Lancet* 7909:740, 1975.

32. Navarro, V. A critique of the present and proposed strategies for redistributing resources in the health sector and a discussion of alternatives. *Medical Care* 12(9): 721–742, 1974.

33. Navarro, V. What does Chile mean? An analysis of the events in the health sector before, during and after Allende's administration. *Health and Society* 52(2): 93–130, 1974. (See also pp. 33–66 of this volume.)

34. Gorz, A. *Strategy for Labor: A Radical Proposal.* Beacon Press, Boston, 1964.

The Underdevelopment of Health
of Working America: Causes,
Consequences and Possible Solutions

To the memory of the Haymarket workers in Chicago, whose struggle in
May 1886 for an eight-hour work day (instead of the fourteen hours
prevalent at that time) became the battle cry of the international workers'
movement, with the establishment of the 1st of May as International Labor
Solidarity Day.

The Rediscovery of a Forgotten Majority—
the Working Class

To the same degree that we in the United States discovered Blacks and
other minorities in the 1960s, and discovered one of our majorities—
women—in the early 1970s, it seems that we are rediscovering in the mid-
70s another forgotten majority—the working class—the members of
which constitute by far the largest sector of both our labor force and our
population. Until very recently, the image of the U.S., perpetuated by
most segments of the media and academia, was that of a middle-class
society, a society in which the majority of our citizens were in the middle
of the social spectrum, and a society in which anyone, if given a chance,
could make it. Indeed, the very category of social class was thought to
have been transcended and made irrelevent by the evolution of social
events. But as Levison (1) and others (2, 3) have shown, the perception of
the U.S. as a middle-class society was more the result of our illusions of
the 1960s than of our realities of the 60s and 70s. Indeed, it is becoming
increasingly clear that we have been, are, and will continue to be for quite
a while a society in which the working class is the majority of our
population. Moreover, most of our minorities (Blacks, Latinos, and other
ethnic groups), as well as the majority of women, are, either by
employment or by association, members of the working class. Social class
and working class, then, are not passé categories in this U.S. of ours, but,
quite to the contrary, are the very core of our realities. Moreover, and as I
will try to show in this presentation, the category of social class is of
paramount importance in understanding the causes and consequences of,
as well as the solutions for, the underdevelopment of the health of our
working population. With this introduction, then, let me briefly (a)

describe the health conditions of the working class, both outside and within the work place, (b) analyze the why of that situation, (c) evaluate the present strategies for change, and (d) present some alternative solutions.

An analysis of the class structure of the U.S. shows that at the top of our society is a relatively small number of people who own a markedly disproportionate share of personal wealth and whose income is largely derived from ownership. While many of these owners also control the use to which their assets are put, this control is increasingly being vested in people who, although wealthy themselves, do not personally own more than a small part of the assets they control—the managers of wealth. Both the owners and controllers of wealth constitute what can be defined as the upper or corporate class, and they command, by virtue of ownership or control or both, the most important sectors of U.S. economic life. At the other end of the social scale is the working class, composed primarily of industrial or blue-collar workers, service workers, and agricultural wage earners, with the latter forming a steadily decreasing proportion of the total labor force.[1] In 1970, these groups represented 35 per cent, 12 per cent, and 1.8 per cent of the labor force, respectively (5, p. 225). This working class remains everywhere a distinct and specific social formation "by virtue of a combination of characteristics which affect its members in comparison with the members of other classes" (4, p. 16). It is also primarily from its ranks that come the unemployed, the poor and the subproletariat.

Between the corporate and working classes is the middle class, consisting of (a) the professionals, including doctors, lawyers, middle-rank executives, academicians, etc., whose main characteristic is that their work is intellectual as opposed to manual and usually requires professional training; (b) the business-middle class, associated with small and medium-sized enterprises, ranging from businessmen employing a few workers to owners of fairly sizeable enterprises of every kind, the owners and controllers of what O'Connor (6, pp. 13–15) has called the competitive sector of our economy; (c) the self-employed shopkeepers, craftsmen and artisans, a declining sector, representing less than 8 per cent of the labor force; and (d) the office and sales workers (the majority of white-collar workers), the group that has increased most rapidly within

[1]In my categorization of classes, I have very closely followed Chapter 2, "Economic Elites and Dominant Classes," in R. Miliband (4, pp. 23–48). It is recognized that this categorization is far from complete. Still, with all its limitations, it is presented in this article as an entry point to our understanding of the composition of the labor force and of the distribution of economic and political power in the U.S.

the labor force in the last two decades and that today represents almost a quarter of that force in the United States and in most Western European countries (7, p. 245). For reasons of brevity, and accepting the simplifications that this categorization implies, I shall refer to groups (a) and (b) as the upper-middle class, and groups (c) and (d) as the lower-middle class. It is worth underlining that the lower-middle class is closely related to the working class with respect to income, status, and life style. For example, most women clerical and sales workers are married, and about one-half are married to working class men (1, pp. 17–53). Figure 1 summarizes the percentage distribution of the labor force by occupational group and sex, and by social class.

We find that close to 80 per cent of the labor force (and approximately 80 per cent of the U.S. population) are members of the lower-middle and working classes, while 20 per cent are members of the upper-middle and corporate classes.

In summary, then, an analysis of the social structure of the United States shows that social classes do indeed exist. Moreover, the analysis of the patterns of ownership of wealth and of the consumption of income shows that both are highly concentrated and that their distribution follows class lines. Indeed, less than 2 per cent of the population—the members of the corporate class and top echelons of the upper-middle class—owns at least 80 per cent of all corporate stocks (the most important type of income-producing wealth) and virtually all state and local government bonds.[2] A similar concentration appears in the distribution of income. In 1971, the working and lower-middle classes, or 80 per cent of the population, consumed 52 per cent of all family personal income, while the corporate and upper-middle classes—20 per cent of the population—consumed 46 per cent (10, pp. 111–136). Thus, we *do* have a class structure in which very few consume and own a great deal and very many, the majority of the U.S. population—the working and lower-middle classes—consume relatively little and own even less.

The Underdevelopment of Health of Working America

Within this social class structure, let us now analyze the picture of health, or lack of it, of our working population. And we find that the picture of

---

[2]These data are from Lampman (8), the most detailed study of individual ownership of wealth ever undertaken in the U.S. Subsequent studies do not indicate any changes in this pattern of ownership. See reference 9, for example.

Figure 1

Occupational, Social Class, and Sex Distribution in the United States

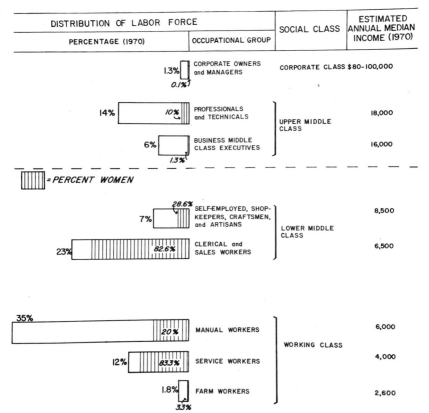

DISTRIBUTION OF LABOR FORCE		SOCIAL CLASS	ESTIMATED ANNUAL MEDIAN INCOME (1970)
PERCENTAGE (1970)	OCCUPATIONAL GROUP		
1.3% 0.1%	CORPORATE OWNERS and MANAGERS	CORPORATE CLASS $80-100,000	
14% 10%	PROFESSIONALS and TECHNICALS	UPPER MIDDLE CLASS	18,000
6% 1.3%	BUSINESS MIDDLE CLASS EXECUTIVES		16,000
= PERCENT WOMEN			
7% 28.6%	SELF-EMPLOYED, SHOP-KEEPERS, CRAFTSMEN, and ARTISANS	LOWER MIDDLE CLASS	8,500
23% 82.6%	CLERICAL and SALES WORKERS		6,500
35% 20%	MANUAL WORKERS	WORKING CLASS	6,000
12% 83.3%	SERVICE WORKERS		4,000
1.8% 3.3%	FARM WORKERS		2,600

Sources: V. Bownell and M. Reich, *Workers and the American Economy: Data on the Labor Force,* New England Free Press, 1973; *Current Population Reports, Consumer Income: Income Growth Rates in 1939 to 1968 for Persons by Occupation and Industry Groups, for the United States,* Series P60, No. 69, 1970; A. Giddens, *The Class Structure of the Advanced Societies,* Hutchinson University Press, 1973.

mortality and morbidity in the U.S. can also be explained in terms of social class. Even if we take income and occupation as indicators of class (and we all know the limitations of these indicators), using age-standardized figures, we find far more mortality and morbidity among the working class than among the corporate and upper-middle classes. For example, in a recent study of mortality by residential patterns in the region of Baltimore, Lerner and Stutz found higher age-standardized mortality among working class communities than among upper class communities, and that this mortality differential has been increasing rather than decreasing in the last thirteen years (11). In terms of morbidity, Conover has shown that nationwide, working class individuals have proportionally more chronic conditions than do members of the upper classes (12). But it is not my intention here to repeat the findings of an increasing number of studies that show that social class is indeed a very important variable in explaining the distribution of disease in our society. I mention these studies to show not only that the category of social class has not been transcended, but also that it is of paramount importance in understanding the distribution of mortality and morbidity in our population, which, to a large degree, follows social class lines.

Any survey of the importance of social class in explaining the distribution of death and disease would be incomplete without considering the mortality and morbidity that is imposed on the working class at the work place. In fact, according to a recent study published by the U.S. Department of Health, Education, and Welfare, there are at least 4 million workers who contract occupational diseases every year, with as many as 100,000 deaths each year (13, pp. 75–162), with the number of deaths in work-related accidents reaching approximately 28,000 (14). The dramatic dimensions of this occupational problem appear increasingly clear for all to see. For example, a recent survey of the working conditions of one-million workers in Chicago carried out by the Bureau of Occupational Safety and Health of the U.S. Department of Health, Education, and Welfare, showed that nearly one-half of them were exposed to "urgent and serious health hazards" on the job (15). And this is just one among many examples of mortality and morbidity imposed on the working population at the work place clearly outlined in a recent article by Arnold Miller, the President of the United Mine Workers of America (16), as well as in the detailed information presented in the chartbook, *Health and Work in America,* prepared for the 1975 annual meeting of the American Public Health Association (17). All these references show that there are indeed many preventable deaths, accidents, and sicknesses that are generated at the work place, the existence of which depicts a callous disregard by our political and economic institutions for the health and safety of our working population.

And as objects of this disregard, two groups merit special mention. One is the coal miners, whose safety conditions are among the poorest in the Western world. On the average, one miner is killed every other day in

U.S. coal mines (18).[3] And 4,000 miners die each year from black lung disease, with one out of every five working miners being a victim of black lung (20). And the second group is the migrant workers, whose life expectancy is forty-nine years, 20 per cent less than that of the average American, and whose infant mortality is 60 per cent above the national average (21). While the scandalous conditions of mortality and morbidity among these two groups are the clearest examples of the death and disease imposed on the majority of our working population at their work place, they are by no means the only ones. Indeed, as A. Miller has indicated, "occupational disease infects this nation like a plague" (16, p. 1218).

Alienation of the Working Population at the Work Place

But there is another component of the occupational situation that is rarely talked about, although it has to do with the nature of work in our society. For the majority of workers, work is not a means of creativity and self-expression, but rather a means of getting the income necessary to participate in the consumer society. Without control over the nature, product, and conditions of their work and denied the opportunity for self-realization at the work place, workers must look for that self-realization and fulfillment in the never-ending sphere of consumption. Thus, work is but a means for that never-achieved satisfaction supposedly to take place via the fetishism of consumption. And that means—work—is beyond the control of the worker, who is alienated and powerless to shape its nature. Despite this reality, the entire concept of worker alienation was dismissed in the 1960s as irrelevant to the actual conditions and perceptions of the working class, and the ubiquitous Gallup Polls, showing that the majority of workers were satisfied with their jobs, seemed to confirm that perception. As Wright and others have shown, however, those results represented more the biases of the researchers than the views of the respondents. When the questions were phrased differently, it appeared that feelings of helplessness, withdrawal, alienation, malaise and pessimism were not minority but majority sentiments among substantial sections of the working class, primarily among younger workers, to such a degree as to become an industrial problem (22). As Walter Dance, Vice President of General Electric, indicated:

[3]For a presentation of mortality and morbidity among coal miners and migrant workers, see reference 19; also included on pp. 67–81 of this volume.

We see a potential problem of vast significance to all industrial companies
. . . This involves the slowly rising feeling of frustration, irritation and
alienation of the blue collar worker, the "hard hats," if you will, but not just
the activists in big cities (quoted in 22, p. ii).

Subsequent studies, such as the report on *Worker Alienation, 1972*
(22) of the Committee on Labor and Public Welfare of the 92nd United
States Congress, show that alienation is prevalent, not only among blue-,
but also white-collar workers. And, as the report of a special task force to
the U.S. Secretary of Health, Education, and Welfare, entitled *Work in
America,* indicates, a main reason for those producers' alienation is the
limiting effect of the nature of their work and their powerlessness to
change it (24).

In summary, creativity and self-fulfillment at the work place are
indeed sacrificed to the almighty efficiency and productivity of Capital,
the actual controller of work and the main controller of our consumer
society. As Sweezy writes in his introduction to H. Braverman's seminal
work, *Labor and Monopoly Capital: The Degradation of Work in the
Twentieth Century:*

> The sad, horrible, heart-breaking way the vast majority of my fellow
> countrymen and women, as well as their counterparts in most of the rest of
> the world, are obliged to spend their working lives is seared into my
> consciousness in an excruciating and unforgettable way. And when I think of
> all the talent and energy which daily go into devising ways and means of
> making their torment worse, all in the name of efficiency and productivity
> but really for the greater glory of the great god Capital, my wonder at
> humanity's ability to create such a monstrous system is surpassed only by
> amazement at its willingness to tolerate the continuance of an arrangement
> so obviously destructive of the well-being and happiness of human beings. If
> the same effort, or only half of it, were devoted to making work the joyous
> and creative activity it can be, what a wonderful world this could be
> (25, p. ix).

And it is the absence of such joy, fulfillment, and control that explains the
overall pervasive feelings of frustration, powerlessness, alienation and
despair among large sectors of our working population.

What Is Being Done?

Having explained the dimensions of the underdevelopment of health in
working America, let us now ask what is being done to correct it. And the
answer, a clear one, is that very little is being done. For example, even

though mining and agricultural work were reported in 1969 by the National Safety Council as being among the most hazardous occupations in terms of deaths and accidents, little progress has been made in determining the extent of the problem, let alone correcting it. In terms of agricultural work, there is not even a national reporting system to record the extent and effect of long-term exposure to pesticides; nor is there a workers' compensation fund to meet claims for medical and unemployment benefits for such workers. And for miners, it was not until 1969 that the first black lung benefits were established; and even today, the amount of money per miner going to study ways of improving safety in the mines and the occupational health among miners is one-twentieth(!) of that spent in the majority of European countries for the same purpose (19). And a similar disregard appears for all other sectors of our working population. Actually, none other than the head of the Occupational Safety and Health Administration (OSHA) of the present Ford administration (not well known, incidentally, as being friendly to Labor), indicated in his keynote address to the 1975 annual meeting of the APHA that not many laws exist to protect the U.S. worker (26). The absence of meaningful legislation to protect our working population is dramatically clear in this example mentioned by A. Miller:

> If a factory worker drives his car recklessly and cripples a factory owner, the worker loses his license to drive, receives a heavy fine, and may spend some time in jail. But, if a factory owner runs his business recklessly and cripples 500 workers with mercury poisoning, he rarely loses his license to do business, and never goes to jail. He may not even have to pay a fine (16, p. 1219).

So much for justice in the U.S.!

The Why of This Situation?

In order to answer the question of why there is such a poor record of protection of the majority of our working force at the work place, we must return to the social class structure of the U.S. and to the understanding of the different degrees of dominance and control that those classes have over the economic, political, and social institutions in our society. In terms of the economic institutions, I have already shown that the majority of the U.S. population owns or controls virtually none of the wealth of our society.

Regarding the political institutions, Figure 2 shows the estimated

Figure 2

Social Class Distribution of the U.S. Labor Force and of the Executive
and Legislative Branches of the U.S. Federal Government

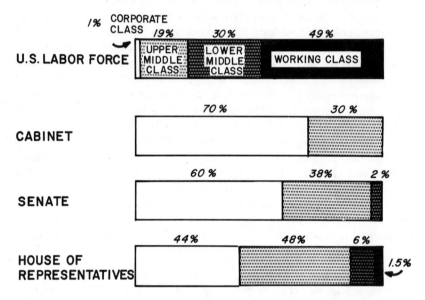

Sources: V. Bownell and M. Reich, *Workers and the American Economy: Data on the Labor Force,* New England Free Press, 1973; A. Giddens, *The Class Structure of the Advanced Societies,* Hutchinson University Press, 1973; M. Barone, G. Ujifusa, and D. Matthews, *The Almanac of American Politics, 1974,* Gambit, 1973.

present class composition of the U.S. labor force and of members of the
U.S. Cabinet, U.S. Senate, and the U.S. House of Representatives.[4] The
corporate class and its dependent upper-middle class, which control most
of the means of production of wealth and legitimation in our society, also
exercise the hegemonic influence over the organs of the state, including
the executive and legislative branches of government.[5] And a similar
pattern of class dominance appears in our social institutions, including
health institutions.

[4]The class structure of political institutions is defined by either the occupation of the
politicians prior to their election or by their association with power blocs, as detailed in
reference 27. Also, see reference 28.

[5]The term "state" includes those institutions—the executive, the legislature, the military and
the police, and the judicial branch—whose interrelationships shape the form of the state
system. For a further expansion of this point, see reference 4.

Let me stress here that the predominance of members of the corporate and upper-middle classes in our political corridors of power is not the cause but rather a symptom of the pattern of class dominance in our society. Also, let me further underline that I do not assume that the corporate class, or any other class for that matter, is uniform or that all its members share the same interests. Indeed, social classes are divided according to power blocs that compete for political influence,[6] and it is this competition that usually passes in our media and academia as the "great U.S. pluralism." But in that competition for political influence, power blocs from the upper-middle class and especially from the corporate class consistently wield far, far more influence over the organs of the state than power blocs belonging to the lower-middle and working classes. As Schattschneider has indicated, "The flaw in the pluralistic heaven is that the heavenly chorus sings with a very special accent . . . the system is askew, loaded, and unbalanced in favor of a fraction of a minority" (30, p. 31). Indeed, underlying and transcending those specific power bloc interests, there are far more important class interests that are paramount in explaining the political behavior of our system. Thus, more frequently than not, federal legislation produces a consistent pattern of effects that benefit the 20 per cent at the top more than the 80 per cent at the bottom of our society. A clear example of this, as O'Connor (6) has shown, is the fiscal and monetary policies of the U.S. government, a most recent example being the effect that the anti-inflationary legislation (approved by the Republican-controlled executive branch of government and passed by the Democrat-controlled Congress) has had on income distribution in this country. As Sylvia Ann Hewlett recently showed in the *New York Times,* a deterioration in levels of income and a widening of inequality between the corporate and executive groups on the one hand and the majority of our population on the other are the most tangible results of anti-inflationary policies of our federal branches of government (31).

In summary, one can see a pattern of consistent and continuous class dominance in our corridors of power in which the few control much and the many very little. And the many know it. Indeed, there is an increasing awareness by the majority of the American people that the political system, for example, does not work for them, but primarily for the few. A recent Harris Poll survey on public attitudes towards government conducted for a U.S. Congressional Committee concludes that

---

[6]For a detailed discussion on this point, see reference 29.

the most striking verdict rendered (in the survey) by the American people—
and disputed by their leaders—is a negative one. A majority of Americans
display a degree of alienation and discontent (with government) . . . (Those)
citizens who thought something was "deeply wrong" with their country had
become a national majority . . . And for the first time in the ten years of
opinion sampling by the Harris Survey, the growing trend of public opinion
toward disenchantment with government swept more than half of all
Americans with it (32, p. vi).

And the nature of that alienation was clearly reflected in the last Hart
Research Associates Poll (33, p. 16–17), which indicated that:

57 per cent of the people agree with the statement that both major parties are
in favor of big business [the code word for corporate class].

58 per cent believe that America's major corporations tend to dominate and
determine the behavior of our public officials in Washington.

50 per cent agree that big business [corporate class] is the source of most of
what is wrong in our society.

It is interesting that in spite of the continuous obfuscation of reality by the
corporate-controlled media and by large sectors of academia, we can see
how our citizenry do contrast that media message with their own realities.
And they are finding that reality increasingly clear to see.

Responses of the System: A Critique of Prevalent Ideologies and Strategies

What are the responses of the system to the social and political realities
presented in the previous sections? An increasingly heard response, and
one advocated by individuals as ideologically diverse as President Ford
and the rebellious Ivan Illich, is that we have to change our life styles and
rely more upon on the individual, i.e. the individual as the ultimate
decider and responsible for his or her choices.[7] And because of its
assumption that the basic cause of our problems is the individual rather
than the economic and political structure of our society, the strategy for
change put forth by adherents of this approach is that of altering our life
styles and public attitudes. In that respect, it is assumed that we, the
people, have been the ones who have chosen our way of living and dying.
And, in a recent book, popular among our corridors of power and
suggestively entitled *Who Shall Live: Health, Economics, and Social*

[7]For a more detailed analysis of this "life-style" strategy, see reference 34.

Choice, the author postulates that we, Americans, have the type of death we deserve and that we have chosen (35). For that author, the logical solution is for the most enlightened leaders and groups to educate our citizens to make better and more rational choices.

Needless to say, this approach is highly popular among the controllers of our system. It continues and replicates the mythology that the economic and political system is basically responsive to what the citizens want. But an analysis of the political behavior of that system shows what a majority of the U.S. population already knows, i.e. that our system is not responsive. For the majority of the U.S. population, the statement that we, the American people, make the social choices and determine the priorities is highly inaccurate. And the fallacy of that statement becomes most clear in the analysis of the underdevelopment of health of our working population. Indeed, to imply that the poor health conditions of our working population shown in this article are the choice of our working population—the majority of our population—is to demonstrate a clear lack of awareness of the distribution of class power in this country, as well as a highly inaccurate understanding of our U.S. reality.

Analysis of Alternatives: The Political Nature of Public Health

Contrary to the prevalent ideologies, I believe that the main health problems of working America are a result of the lack of power and control over our economic, political and social institutions by the majority of our population.

In that respect, I would encourage you to think of social medicine and public health not only in terms of improving water and sewage systems, or even in terms of improving occupational medicine, but also and primarily (as did the founders of social medicine) in terms of redistributing the economic and political power in our society from a few to the many. Indeed, Virchow, the founder of social medicine, clearly saw the need to merge the medical task with the political and social forces that were mobilized by the emerging working class. Virchow, who joined the first working class revolt of March 18, 1848 in his own city of Berlin and who also supported the workers' rebellion against the French bourgeoisie in the Paris Commune, clearly saw our task as being political. And in his writings on public health, he concluded that

that very word Public Health shows those who were and still are of the
opinion that medicine has nothing to do with politics the magnitude of their
error.

Moreover, he added that "Medicine is a social science and politics is
medicine on a large scale" (quoted in 36, p. 62). It could not have been
said better. Actually, there is a real need to stress over and over again the
political nature of our tasks, since there are powerful conservative forces
that want to "depoliticize" public health and present our problems as
merely managerial and technological ones. And we are told that in a
technological society, supposedly the most "unideological" of all societies,
all problems can be reduced to managerial problems, i.e. that our task is a
value-free, neutral one. But several social events in our society, from the
antiwar movement to the recent nationwide coal-miners' strike, show that
ours is a conflictive society with a daily battle of ideologies, and that ours
is a political task in which the illusion of being neutral is an indicator of
being on the wrong side.

According to this interpretation, most of our public health problems
are political problems and thus most of our solutions are political
solutions. Therefore, the greatest need for all progressive forces in the
U.S. today is to create the political movement that can represent the
desire for control by the working population of its resources and
institutions. Actually, it is interesting to note that according to the Hart
Poll mentioned above, *the majority of the public favors employee
ownership and control of U.S. companies—not worker participation, but
control—with local communities represented on the boards of companies
that operate in their local regions* (33). The implications of that popular
belief are enormous. But, in spite of this, and as we would expect, not one
politician in the U.S. Congress has as much as suggested any type of
legislation that even begins to reflect this reality.

In the absence of any meaningful demand by either of the two major
political parties in this country for major changes in the distribution of
economic and political power, I suggest there is a need to develop a
political movement that can link and organize that popular feeling for
control of our political, economic, and social institutions. And a primary
condition for that task is to develop the awareness that the different
groups and causes that exist on our progressive horizons have more
things in common than against. As one foreign observer indicated
recently, we in the U.S. have too many liberation movements and not
enough of a Liberation Movement. We need to establish the political
links among all progressive causes that can unite their strength rather

than divide it. If political maturity is the capacity to relate things in our political system, then we need to develop that mature political movement that can embrace and relate all of the different progressive causes and that can link those separate movements without stifling them.

Another urgent task in the development of such a political movement is to rediscover the history of our country. The progressive forces in this country are far too divided, divided according to their support for too many foreign models. There is a need to transcend being pro-Soviet, pro-Cuban, pro-Chinese, or pro-whatever, and be instead pro-U.S.; not the U.S. of the corporate class, but the U.S. of the majority of our population—the working population. And a first condition for this is to rediscover the history of the working class of this country, a history of long and hard class struggle. For example, very few people seem to realize that the famous 1st of May started in this country, in Chicago, in honor of those who died in the Haymarket strike in the struggle for the eight-hour work day, and was later chosen by the international socialist movement as a day of international socialist solidarity (37). And very few people know that the Labor Day weekend was established by the then corporate-class-controlled U.S. Congress as a substitute for May Day, as a way of quieting and supplanting that international workers' solidarity.

There is indeed a need to rediscover the history of the U.S. and establish a link with that historical past which will enable a rediscovery of the working class and its history, and to build upon it a working class movement that will come from the working class itself.

Let me emphasize here that a sense of history is also unfortunately absent in the public health movement. Few young health workers realize that large sectors of that movement had been socialist in the past and that those workers and their leaders suffered oppression and repression in the nefarious McCarthy era (still existent today) because of their beliefs. It was that repression that either left them emotionally exhausted and/or forced them to keep a low political profile. To them I want to pay tribute and extend the invitation to come out and show their own true colors. Indeed, I believe that it is time for socialists to get out of the closet! They represent an experience that is much needed and with which there is an urgency to establish a continuity. The future cannot be built without the foundations of the past. But to build on the past does not mean to repeat the past. New strategies for change need to be developed that go beyond past strategies. For example, the classical categories of debate on private versus public ownership need to be transcended. There *is* a need for public control of our major resources, and the American public is ready for it. Again, according to that Hart Poll (33), the majority of U.S. citizens believe that oil companies, for example, should be nationalized. And it is interesting that in spite of this, not one politician has made such a proposal in our Congress.

But public ownership is not answer enough. Our American public has a justified concern about big government being an oppressive rather than liberating force. Thus, there is a need to underline that public control has to mean the public's control of our resources, i.e. control of our resources and of our institutions by the individuals working in them and by the communities served by them. And proposals are appearing in each sector of our life that respond to that demand. Specifically, in the health sector, proposals are being made based on worker and community control (38). Calls for such control to take place in our society will no doubt be dismissed by many as merely Utopian. But to this, we must answer that we perceive our task as one of making Utopia believable, credible, and accessible to our population. As Marcuse has indicated, the ideological success of our capitalist system has been to make the possibility of alternatives unthinkable. But it is the task of the authentically progressive forces in this country to make those alternatives both thinkable and feasible—and not for the distant future when socialism comes, but for now, today, in the very womb of capitalism. And what we hear from the majority of our population shows that they are far more ready for that than many of us seem to realize.

In summary, I perceive the public health task as serving and supporting the public's demands not only for health resources, but also for control of those and all resources that they produce. But in order to undertake that task, it is necessary to realize that we cannot have a progressive health movement in the absence of a progressive political movement. It is to the establishment of that broader movement the public health workers should also give utmost priority. And it should be stressed over and over again that the development of health requires not managerial, but political changes aimed at a most profound change of our society—to break with the control by the few over the many. And consequently, our commitment to the public's health, to the health of our people, demands our political commitment to democratize our society authentically, with a degree of redistribution of economic and political power far, far more profound than is envisioned in any of the current political alternatives put forth by the two major political forums in our country. In summary, then, there is a need to link the public health struggles, both at the local and national levels, with larger political struggles at all levels—political struggles that should be aimed at profoundly transforming a system that works primarily for the few and not for the many. The production of freedom and democracy and the production of health are indeed the same.

References

1. Levison, A. *The Working Class Majority.* Coward, McCann, and Geoghegan, Inc., New York, 1974.

2. Parker, R. *The Myth of the Middle Class.* Liveright, New York, 1972.

3. Szymanski, A. Trends in the American class structure. *Socialist Revolution* 10:101–122, 1972.

4. Miliband, R. *The State in Capitalist Society: An Analysis of the Western System of Power.* Weidenfeld and Nicolson, London, 1969.

5. U.S. Bureau of the Census. *Statistical Abstract of the United States: 1970.* U.S. Government Printing Office, Washington, D.C., 1970.

6. O'Connor, J. *The Fiscal Crisis of the State.* St. Martin's Press, New York, 1973.

7. Dahrendorf, R. Recent changes in the class structure of European societies. *Daedalus,* Winter, 1964.

8. Lampman, R.J. *The Share of Top Wealth-Holders in National Wealth, 1922–1956.* Princeton University Press, Princeton, N.J., 1956.

9. Upton, L. and Lyons, N. *Basic Facts: Distribution of Personal Income and Wealth in the U.S.* Cambridge Institute, Cambridge, Mass., 1972.

10. Miller, H.P. Income distribution in the United States, in Atkinson, A.B. (ed.). *Wealth, Income, and Inequality.* Penguin, London, 1973.

11. Lerner, M. and Stutz, R.N. *Mortality Differentials Among Socio-Economic Strata in Baltimore, 1960 and 1973.* 1975 Social Statistics Section, Proceedings of the American Statistical Association (in press).

12. Conover, P.W. Social class and chronic illness. *International Journal of Health Services* 3:357–368, 1973

13. Discher, D.P., et al. *Pilot Study for Development of an Occupational Disease Surveillance Method.* National Institute for Occupational Safety and Health, U.S. Department of Health, Education, and Welfare. U.S. Government Printing Office, Washington, D.C., 1975.

14. Gordon, J.B., Ackman, A. and Brooks, M.L. *Industrial Safety Statistics: A Re-examination: A Critical Report Prepared for the U.S. Dept. of Labor.* Praeger Publishers, New York, 1971.

15. Bureau of Occupational Safety and Health, U.S. Department of Health, Education, and Welfare. *Occupational Health Survey of the Chicago Metropolitan Area.* U.S. Government Printing Office, Washington, D.C., 1970.

16. Miller, A. The wages of neglect: death and disease in the American work place. *American Journal of Public Health* 65: 1217–1220, 1975.

17. *Health and Work in America: A Chart Book.* American Public Health Association, Washington, D.C., 1975.

18. Research Unit, United Mine Workers of America. Written Communication to the Author, 1975.

19. Navarro, V. The political and economic determinants of health and health care in rural America. *Inquiry* 13(2):111–121, 1976. (See also pp. 67–81 of this volume.)

20. Shoub, E.B. *Overview of Coalminers' Health Findings.* Sixth Annual Institute of Coal Mining Health, Safety and Research, Virginia Polytechnic Institute and State University, Blacksburg, Virginia, August 27, 1975.

21. Senate Subcommittee on Migratory Labor, U.S. Congress. Hearings on Migratory Labor. U.S. Government Printing Office, Washington, D.C., 1972.

22. Senate testimony by James Wright, Director, National Policy Affairs, National Center for Urban Ethnic Affairs. In *Worker Alienation, 1972.* Hearings before the Subcommittee on Employment, Manpower, and Poverty of the Committee on Labor and Public Welfare, United States Senate, 92nd Congress, pp. 29–35. U.S. Government Printing Office, Washington, D.C., 1972.

23. Sheppard, H.L. and Herrick, N.Q. *Where Have All the Robots Gone? Worker Dissatisfaction in the 70s.* Free Press, New York, 1972.

24. Report of a Special Task Force to the Secretary of H.E.W. *Work in America.* M.I.T. Press, Cambridge, Mass., 1973.

25. Sweezy, P.M. In foreword to Braverman, H. *Labor and Monopoly Capital: The Degradation of Work in the Twentieth Century.* Monthly Review Press, New York, 1974.

26. Corn, M. Health and work in America. Keynote Address, 103rd Annual Meeting of the American Public Health Association, Chicago, November 17, 1975.

27. Barone, M., Ujifusa, G. and Matthews, D. *The Almanac of American Politics: The Senators, The Representatives, Their Records, States and Districts, 1974.* Gambit, Boston, 1974.

28. Lyons, R.D. Records show 22 millionaires in House. *New York Times,* p. 42, January 4, 1976.

29. Poulantzas, N. *Classes in Contemporary Capitalism.* New Left Review Editions, London, 1975.

30. Schattschneider, E.E. *The Semi-Sovereign People: A Realistic View of Democracy in America.* Holt, Rinehart and Winston, New York, 1960.

31. Hewlett, S.A. Inflation and inequality. *New York Times,* October 24, 1974.

32. Committee on Government Operations, United States Senate. *Confidence and Concern: Citizens View American Government: A Survey of Public Attitudes, Part 1.* U.S. Government Printing Office, Washington, D.C., 1973.

33. Complete Hart Poll Results, published in *Common Sense.* September 1, 1975.

34. Navarro, V. The industrialization of fetishism or the fetishism of industrialization: a critique of Ivan Illich. *Social Science and Medicine* 9: 351–363, 1975. Also included on pp. 103–131 of this volume.

35. Fuchs, V. *Who Shall Live: Health, Economics and Social Choice.* Basic Books, New York, 1975.

36. Rosen, G. *From Medical Police to Social Medicine: Essays in the History of Health Care.* Neale Watson Publications, New York, 1974.

37. Yellen, S. *American Labor Struggles.* Arno Press, New York, 1969.

38. Summary of National Health Rights and Community Health Services Act. *Congressional Record,* Vol. 121, No. 49. U.S. Government Printing Office, Washington, D.C., 1975.

PART II:
THE MEANING OF HEALTH
AND MEDICINE

The Industrialization of Fetishism:
A Critique of Ivan Illich

According to the media and other organs of popularization, our Western developed societies are in crisis. Thus, the number of analysts and synthesizers providing remedies to this crisis is proliferating. One of them is Ivan Illich, Director of the Centre for Intercultural Documentation in Cuernavaca, Mexico. Widely quoted and debated, he has been variously defined as the genius who provides the focus for our doubts (1), a revolutionary who gives the best prescription for change (2), and a "petit réactionnaire" who is nostalgically looking for Bucolia (3). But whatever characterization may best apply to Illich, he is an articulate theoretician and one of the more recent in a long roster of builders of what I consider to be the most prevalent and influential ideology used to explain our societies, i.e. the ideology of industrialism. As such, his work merits serious response.

Assuming that the best way to understand an author's analysis of our reality is by first comprehending the ideological framework on which that analysis is based, let me begin by summarizing very briefly the main characteristics of the ideology of industrialism of which Illich's writings are part and parcel. I will then describe how those characteristics appear both in his analysis of our Western developed societies and of our health services as well as in his normative synthesis, i.e. the basis for his strategy for change. In both cases the main, but not only, point of reference will be Illich's most recent book, *Medical Nemesis* (4).[1] In the second part of this article I will discuss the assumptions underlying Illich's ideology and will analyze the degree to which they provide valid explanations of the actual situation in our Western developed countries and in our health services. Where the explanations are found to be invalid, I will present alternate explanations of the social problematique of our countries. And in the third part, in light of those alternative explanations, I will discuss the extent to which Illich's recommendations for change are relevant to the solution of our problems.

[1]This book has been briefly summarized in the *Lancet* (5) and in *Social Policy* (6). Unless otherwise indicated, the references to Illich's *Medical Nemesis* are to the book (4) and not to its summaries.

Industrialism As Ideology and Its Presentation in Illich's Writings

Industrialism is the most prevalent ideology used to explain the nature and form of our Western developed societies. Grounded largely in technological determinism it owes much to Max Weber, and it suggests that the industrial nature of technology defines social organizations in their entirety (7).

Among the primary characteristics of that ideology is that the production requirements of the technological process and, pari passu of industrial organizations, are the most important determinants of the nature and form of our Western developed societies, i.e. industrialized societies. In a fatalistic and almost deterministic way the former—the technological process—leads inevitably to the latter—the industrialization of society. Moreover, according to the theorists of industrialism, that industrialization has transcended and made irrelevant and passé the categories of property, ownership, and social class. Indeed, ownership loses its meaning as legitimization of power. And control, now assumed to be divorced from ownership, has passed from the owners of capital— the capitalists—to the managers of that capital, and from there to the technocrats, those who have the skills and knowledge needed to operate the major social edifices of industrialism, the bureaucracies. The new elite, then, are the bureaucrats, who have supplanted the capitalists. Within this evolution, a new social order based on bureaucracy has transcended the capitalist order. Capitalist societies have thus become industrial, post-industrial, and mixed-economies societies. As Frankenberg (8) has indicated, words such as capitalism, social class, and related ones rarely pass through these theoreticians' typewriter keys, except in an introductory note of dismissal.

Also, according to the theoreticians of this ideology, in this evolutionary process of industrialization, there is a disintegration of the old preindustrial order, assumed to be integrated, self-sufficient, and communal. In the words of Illich (4, p. 65), because of industrial growth "social arrangements allowing such autonomy [of community members] have practically disappeared." And in the industrial order that replaces it only the values that are functional for the "formal rationality" of the system are sustained and replicated; productivity, efficiency, progress, and modernization are the components of the intellectual-philosophical construct of the ideological building of industrialism. Basic requirements of that construct are the need for hierarchy and dependency within those hierarchies. At the top of that hierarchy is the expert, the bureaucrat; at the bottom is the subject of that bureaucracy, the receiver or consumer of the goods, commodities, or services administered by that bureaucracy. Within this hierarchy the former manipulates the latter, in theory for the benefit of both, in practice for the benefit of the former more than the latter.

A final characteristic of industrialism is that it claims to be a universal process. In other words, all societies, regardless of their political structure, will evolve according to the dictates of industrialization. Indeed, according to a key component of that ideology, *the theory of convergence,* all societies will progress toward the urban-industrial model of the future. Thus, socialism and capitalism are usually seen as two convergent roads to the same destination, "the industrial model." In the words of one of its most successful popularizers (9):

> Such reflection on the future would also emphasize the convergent tendencies of industrial societies, however different their *popular or ideological billing,* the convergence being to a roughly similar design for organization and planning. . . . Convergence begins with modern large-scale production, with heavy requirements of capital, sophisticated technology, and, as a prime consequence, elaborate organization [emphasis added].

The ideologists of industrialism then, including Illich, predict the inevitable development of societies of a unitary type, leading to an urban-industrialized model. In that respect, the history of the human race is the history of the different stages of development toward that model. Accordingly, the degree of development of any country is measured by the extent to which it approximates that model, with the United States being held as the most developed country, i.e. closest to that model.[2]

Viewed in this way, the social problems of society (the U.S.) become not the problems of capitalism (an altogether passé category), but the problems of industrialization. And I tend to suspect that the great prevalence of that ideology throughout our society, including academia, can be explained partially by its self-flattering interpretation of our problems, i.e. the social problems we face result from our pioneering the great search for modernization, and from being ahead in our industrialization. Ours, in summary, is the burden of the leaders. In the words of an

[2]The most representative proponent of this stage theory is Rostow (10). For a critique of Rostow's stages with special emphasis on their implications in the health sector, see reference 11. See also pages 3–32 of this volume. Another work that presents this model is that of Kahn and Wiener (12), in which the level of development of the countries is measured by the estimated number of years that it will take for those countries to reach the 1965 U.S. level of overall economic development, measured by the ubiquitous gross national product per capita.

influential popularizer in the U.S., "We have to pay the social investment of being the first. Others will learn from our failures and successes" (13).

If one accepts this ideology, it then makes sense to study and analyze the social problematique of the already industrialized societies, primarily of the U.S., to see how much other less developed countries can learn from both their successes and failings. Ivan Illich, director of one academic center physically situated in a developing country, Mexico, focuses the attention of all his writings on the industrialized societies, with greatest emphasis on the U.S. Consequently, he draws most of his references from and bases most of his categories on Western developed countries.

If there is general agreement among the theoreticians of industrialism, at least on the main assumptions summarized above, there is far less agreement on the conclusions they draw. Indeed, while some like Daniel Bell (14) and Walt Rostow (10) rejoice over the fruits of industrialization, others like Raymond Aron (15) seem to have second thoughts, and others still, such as Illich (16), despair and try to rebel. Unless we reverse industrialization, writes Illich (5, p. 921), ours will be a "compulsory survival in a planned and engineered Hell." Not surprisingly, then, their suggestions for change differ widely. But an approach increasingly heard, and one that Illich seems to share, can be defined as that of Jeffersonian republicanism which recommends (a) the debureaucratization of our society; (b) the reversal of industrialization and growth with the breaking down of professional and other monopolies toward a return to the free market of goods and services; and (c) a renewed emphasis on the self-reliance and autonomy of the individual, with enlightened self-interest as the prime mover in his relationships of exchange.

Industrialism in Illich's Writings

The ideology of industrialism, placing the credit and in Illich's case the blame for our social development and its problematique on the inevitable process of industrialization, underlies the theoretical constructs used by most analysts of our Western society, including its critics, such as Illich.

Indeed, Illich believes that industrialism is the main force shaping our societies and that unavoidable "rising irreparable damage accompanies industrial expansion in all sections" (5, p. 920), including medicine (4), education (17), and so on. For example, the industrialization of medicine leads to the creation of a corps of engineers—the medical profession—comparable to the technocrats of the main social formation of industrialized societies, the bureaucracy. Thus, the industrialization of medicine means its professionalization and bureaucratization. Moreover, and reflecting the assumed universality claimed by the ideology of industrialism, Illich believes that all societies, either capitalist or socialist, converge toward the same model, following a similar evolutionary process. Indeed, "the frustrations [due to industrialization] which have become manifest from private-enterprise systems and from socialized care have come to resemble each other frighteningly" (5, p. 921). The same problematique that appears in Houston is likely to appear in Moscow, in Bogata to appear in Havana, and in Taiwan to appear in People's China as well. The differences in the expression of that problematique are more quantitative, depending on the level of industrialization and stage of development of those countries, than qualitative. Capitalism and socialism are indeed outmoded concepts, since they are basically converging toward the same path of industrialization that overwhelms and directs their social formations.

In this interpretation, then, the class conflict has been replaced by the conflict between those at the top, the managers of the bureaucracies, indispensable to the running of an industrialized society, and those at the bottom, the consumers of the products—goods and services— administered by those bureaucracies. As applied specifically to medicine, that conflict is the one between the medical bureaucracy, primarily the medical profession and the medical care system, and the consumers, the patients. This antagonistic conflict appears as iatrogenesis (damage done by the provider), and it is

> clinical, when pain, sickness, and death result from the provision of medical care; it is social, when health policies reinforce an industrial organization which generates dependency and ill health; and it is structural, when medically sponsored behaviour and delusions restrict the vital autonomy of people by undermining their competence in growing up, caring for each other and aging (4, p. 165).

The first and most documented type of iatrogenesis is the clinical one, damage done by the physicians and providers of services, and is caused primarily by their engineering approach to medicine in which the individual is seen as a machine, an aggregate of different pieces that have to be put right through therapeutic intervention. Adding to that cause, there is also much injury that is due simply to much arrogance, sheer incompetence, and misunderstanding of what health is about (4, pp. 15–25).

Social iatrogenesis is the addictive dependency of the populace on the medical care institutions. Indeed,

> public [demand and] support for a nationwide addiction to therapeutic relationships is pathogenic on a much deeper level, but this is usually not recognized. More health damages are caused by the belief of people that they cannot cope with illness without modern medicines than by doctors who foist their ministrations on patients (4, p. 39).

In that respect,

> the proliferation of medical institutions, no matter how safe and well engineered, unleashes a social pathogenic process. Over-medicalization changes adaptive ability into passive medical consumer discipline (4, p. 39).

According to Illich, the cause for that addiction is the manipulative behavior of the medical bureaucracy that perpetuates and encourages that passive and addictive consumer behavior. In this scheme of things the power of that bureaucracy is its exclusive and monopolistic power of definition of what is health and what method of care may be publicly funded.

Last but certainly not least, *structural iatrogenesis* is the loss of autonomy of the patient and the creation of his dependency. In this iatrogenesis, the medical bureaucracy goes further than creating addiction, and destroys "the potential of people to deal with their human weakness, vulnerability and uniqueness in a personal and autonomous way" (4, pp. 87–150). According to Illich, the responsibility for health and care is taken away—expropriated—from the individual by the medical industry. Moreover, this structural iatrogenesis is assumed to be intrinsic in the values and modus operandi of the medical industry and civilization. Thus the intervention of the medical industry has the same effect as that of any other industry, i.e. it breaks with those social values and cultures, such as acceptance of death, disease, and pain, assumed to be in existence in the preindustrial societies and that are capable of providing the self-realization of the individual (4, p. 160).

Illich's Strategies for Change: The Debureaucratization and Deindustrialization of Society and Medicine

How can we avoid and correct these iatrogeneses, the extensive damage done by the industrialization of medicine? Before stating his own solutions, Illich briefly considers several other alternatives presently debated in the political scene. In discussing solutions for *clinical* and *social iatrogeneses,* he especially rejects the "socialization alternative" that he attributes to the "equalizing rhetoric" of the misleadingly called progressive forces, among which he includes liberals and Marxists. According to his normative conclusion, the redistribution of medical care implied in the socialization alternative would make matters even worse since it would tend to further medicalize our population and create further dependencies on medical care (4, p. 66). Indeed, "less access to the present health system would, contrary to political rhetoric, benefit the poor" (4, p. 73). In that respect, Illich finds the creation of the National Health Service in Britain as a regressive, not progressive, step.

Instead of socialization and its implied redistribution, Illich recommends the following solutions for clinical and social iatrogeneses:

- The mode of production in medicine should be changed via its deprofessionalization and debureaucratization to break down the barriers that allow the "disbursement of any such public funds under the prescription and control of guild members" (4, p. 121). In that respect he suggests what Friedman (18) and Kessel (19, 20) have proposed in this country—that licensing and regulation of healers should disappear, and the concerns of where, when, how, and from whom to receive care should be left to the choice of the individual.

- Collective responsibility for that care should be reduced and individual responsibility should be maximized. Self-discipline, self-interest, and self-care should be the guiding principles for the individual in maintaining his health. In summary each one should be made responsible for his own health. Indeed, Illich's dictum in health sounds very close to the dictum of another theoretician of the virtue of self-reliance, ex-President Nixon's "don't ask what the state can do for you, but what can you do for yourself" (21).

As to structural iatrogenesis, the most important of the three, and the one that Illich especially attributes to industrialism, he again dismisses the alternative of the socialization and public control of the process of industrialization, recommending instead the reversal of that process, i.e. breaking down the centralization of industry and returning to the market model. According to Illich, "Only the inversion of society's overall growth rate in marketed goods and services can permit a reversal" (4, p. 160). And within this competitive market model, the motivations for social interaction will be those of enlightened self-interest and a desire for survival (4, p. 164). The essence of his strategy for correcting structural iatrogenesis, then, is an anti-trust approach with strong doses not of Marx, or even Keynes, but of Friedman.

A Critique of Illich and an Exploration of Alternatives

Clinical Iatrogenesis: The Illusion of Doctors' Effectiveness

Perhaps not surprisingly, most of the debate on Illich's writings on medicine has focused on his postulate that individual clinical intervention may be doing more harm than good (clinical iatrogenesis). Actually, not only medical journals such as the *Lancet* in Britain, but popular magazines like *Le Nouvel Observateur* in France have focused primarily on Illich's skepticism about the therapeutic value of medical intervention. In this skepticism he follows the by now well established and known tradition of non-medical writers such as Montesquieu, Tolstoy, Bernard Shaw, and many others who have questioned the effectiveness of the professionals' tasks throughout the passing of decades. Unfortunately, the medical profession has dismissed too frequently and too uncritically those questions as being too perverse and frivolous to merit serious considera-tion. And the inquiring minds within the profession that kept asking the same questions and providing evidence to support such skepticisms were and still are equally dismissed or boycotted as unwelcome prophets of an unwelcome change. (For a further discussion of this point see reference 22.)

Illich, in a short but meaningful review of what he defines as the effectiveness of medical care, summarizes the available information on the effectiveness of some therapeutic interventions, and thus provides evidence on the limitations of those interventions. Not unexpectedly, he is more pessimistic about the value of those interventions than most clinicians would be, but paradoxically is far more optimistic about the effectiveness of some of those interventions, e.g. skin cancer treatment or early surgical intervention for cervical cancer (4, pp. 16–19), than most health care researchers would be. (See, for example, reference 23.)

Still, he adds his iconoclastic voice (a welcome voice, I might add) to an increasing chorus of doubters of the effectiveness of medical tasks. A major weakness of his evaluation, however, is that he takes as an indicator of the effectiveness of medical *care,* indicators of *cure.* Indeed, he seems to confuse care with cure. And in evaluating the effectiveness of medical care he does what most clinicians—Illich's engineers in the medical system—do; he analyzes the degree to which medical intervention has reduced mortality and morbidity, i.e. the effectiveness of health care intervention in *curing* disease and avoiding mortality. But, at a time when the most important type of morbidity in our Western developed societies is chronic, a much better indicator of the effectiveness of the medical *care* intervention would be the way that care is provided in that intervention, i.e. the degree to which the system provides supportive and attentive care to those in need. And the limited evidence available does seem to indicate that medical *care* may make a difference, i.e. it may reduce disability and discomfort in people's lives. (For a sketchy review of this *care* effectiveness, see reference 24.) But for that taking *care* to occur, our medical care system would have to change very profoundly to better enable the system to provide that care.

Still, since Illich seems to see an inevitable progress toward the present cure-oriented system, he does not seem to accept the possibility of creating another system in which the priorities would be opposite to those of the present ones, with emphasis given to care as opposed to cure services. Actually, Illich would not even welcome such a care-oriented system since it would increase the dependency of the individual on the physician and on the system of medical care, preventing the much needed self-reliance and autonomy. Indeed, according to Illich, whatever good medical cure or care may do is certainly outbalanced by the damage that it creates. And he finds the greatest damage to be the dependency that medical care creates in the population, i.e. social iatrogenesis.

Social Iatrogenesis: Addiction to Medical Care Institutions, Cause or Symptom?

Illich considers social iatrogenesis, the addictive behavior of the population to medical care, to be the result of manipulation by the medical bureaucracy—the medical care system. It is a manipulation that aims at creating dependency and consumption. Indeed, Illich postulates that the consumer behavior of our citizenry is primarily determined by its manipulation by the bureaucracies created as a result of industrialization. Allow me to focus on this postulate, and to discuss the consumer behavior of our citizenry, not only in the health sector of our economy but in all others as well. Disagreeing with Illich, I find that manipulation of addiction and consumption by bureaucracies (including the medical care bureaucracy) is not the cause, as he postulates, but the symptom of the basic needs of the economic and social institutions of what he calls industrialized societies, but what I would call industrialized capitalist societies.[3] Actually, I consider those bureaucracies, be they trade, services, or "whatever," to be the mere socialization instruments of those needs, i.e. they reinforce and capitalize on what is *already* there—*the need for consumption,* consumption that reflects a dependency of the individual on something that can be bought, either a pill, a drug, a prescription, a car, or the "prepackaged moon." Indeed, the overall quantum of citizens' dependency is far more than the mere aggregate of dependencies of those citizens on the bureaucracies of our societies. Actually, those dependencies are mere symptoms of a more profound dependency that has been created in our citizenry not by industrialization, but by the capitalist mode of production and consumption—a mode of production that results in the majority of men and women in our societies having no control over the product of their work, and a mode of consumption in which the citizenry is directed and manipulated in their consumption of the products of that work. (For excellent reports on how the values are being shaped in our societies, see references 26–28.) As Marcuse (29) has indicated, that system makes people aspire to more when this more must always be inaccessible. This dependency on consumption—this commodity fetishism—is intrinsically necessary for the survival of a system that is based on commodity production. It is then necessary for the owners and controllers of the means of production of that system to stimulate dissatisfaction and dependency in the sphere of consumption. Thus, those owners and controllers must provoke continual artificial dissatisfactions and dependencies in human beings that direct them toward further consumption because without them the system would collapse. And, as I will try to show later, Illich's bureaucracies, including the medical bureaucracies, are not the generators, but the administrators of those dependencies, consumptions, and dissatisfactions. Indeed, those bureaucracies are not the owners nor the controllers, but the administrators of that system.

In summary, in this alternate explanation, addiction and dependency on consumption—either of goods or services—are not due primarily to the manipulative behavior of bureaucracies, but result from the basic needs of an economic system that requires for its survival (a) the creation of wants, however artificial or absurd they may be, (b) the existence of a

[3]In this article capitalist societies are societies in which, notwithstanding the existence of a "public sector," the largest majority of economic activity is still dominated by private ownership and enterprise that primarily benefits a dominant class. In those societies, the state owns only a subsidiary part of the means of production. As Miliband (25) writes, to speak of "mixed economies" in those societies is to attribute a special and quite misleading meaning to the notion of mixture.

passive and "massified" population of consumers, and (c) the replication of consumer ideology whereby the citizen is judged not by what he *does* (his work) but by what he *has* (his consumption). Within that system, the citizen, the consumer, is made to believe that his fulfillment depends in large degree on his consumption, be it of drugs, pills, prescriptions, cosmetics, and whatever else may be required for his fitness, well-being, and pursuit of happiness. Within this scheme of things, to consider that need for consumption, that addictive behavior, to be the result of bureaucratic manipulation is (a) to underestimate the needs of the economic system, and (b) to far overestimate the role of those bureaucracies. Theirs is, again, the task of administering and reinforcing that dependency on consumption that is *already there.*

Let me underline here that I do not deny the powerful effect that Illich's bureaucracies, such as the medical and related bureaucracies, e.g. drug advertising, have on administering and reinforcing (but not creating) a harmful demand for their goods and services. But I don't believe that the disappearance of those bureaucracies (if it were at all possible) from our capitalist societies would mean the disappearance of that addictive demand. Indeed, Illich's focus on the world of consumption and his theories of manipulation ignore the main determinants of people's behavior, which are not in the sphere of consumption, but in the world of production.[4] Indeed, in our capitalist system what the individual might have (defined in the area of consumption) depends on what he might do (defined in the world of production). Indeed, whatever he can buy depends very much on how much money he makes. And for the great majority of our citizens, the amount of money they make depends primarily on what type of work they do and how much they are paid for it. Thus, to understand the *sphere of consumption* we have to understand the *world of production,* or who does what, who controls that work, and how that control takes place. And an analysis of that world of production shows the following: (a) The great majority of producers—the workers— do not have much control over the nature and product of their work. What they do in the workplace and how they do it is, in the great majority of cases, outside the control of the workers, and within the control of the employer. (b) Work is for the majority of producers primarily not a means of self-expression, where creativity is the goal, but a means to get income to be able to buy the services and goods necessary to satisfy their needs. The most important components in one's life, creativity and

---

[4]Also, Illich's focus on the addictive part of medical care consumption seems to ignore a valid need for medical care responsive to the needs for both cure and care of our population.

worthiness, are not realized in one's daily work. In other words, the worker must spend time at work to get freedom and capacity for development outside the sphere of production. Ironically, this hope for fulfillment during leisure time turns out to be an illusion, an illusion that has to be satisfied with the always unsatisfied and never-ending consumption. In summary, denied of his self-realization at his place of work, the world of production, the worker then has to look for that realization in the sphere of consumption. The alienation of the producer from his work—his dissatisfaction—leads to the fetishism of consumption. (For an elaboration of the concept of alienation, see references 30, 31 and 32.) And that alienation determines and creates the feelings of helplessness, malaise and pessimism which, as indicated in the preceding article, are prevalent among large sectors of our working population.

The response to that situation—the alienating effect of work—varies depending on the degree of awareness and consciousness of the individual to that situation. And, one increasingly important response is the expression of that dissatisfaction in labor conflicts. Actually, the number of working days lost in the U.S. due to labor strikes concerning issues of working conditions—the nature of work—exceeds those concerning the size of the paycheck or the amount of fringe benefits (33). (For an excellent account of the alienation of the working class, the majority of the U.S. population, see "The Discontent of Work," in reference 34.)

Another reaction to that alienation is, as Dreitzel (35) has pointed out, its internalization, appearing as a major cause of psychosomatic illness, the type of problem most frequently presented to the medical care system. Indeed,

> doctors from various industrialized countries unanimously report that at least 50 per cent of their patients suffer from "functional disturbances," i.e. illness without any establishable organic cause (37, p. viii).

Thus, in the medical care system we also find that (a) the alienation of the individual in his world of production leads him to the sphere of consumption, the consumption of health services, and that (b) the medical care bureaucracy is just administering those disturbances created by the nature of work and the alienating nature of our system of production. Actually, the increasing awareness of this phenomenon explains the choice by the American Public Health Association of "Work and Health in the U.S." as the main theme for its 1975 Annual Meeting. As an editorial of the journal of that Association (36) indicates, work is the keynote, not only of the restoration of health but also of the maintenance of health in our society. Actually, that editorial repeats what Albert Camus wrote somewhat more elegantly, "Without work all life goes rotten. But when work is soulless, life stifles and dies" (quoted in 37, p. xx).

In summary, Illich's focus on consumption leads him to believe that the loss of autonomy (including the expropriation of his health) and subsequent dependency of the individual are due to the manipulation and effect of the bureaucracies in the individual's sphere of consumption. Disagreeing with him, I believe that the loss of autonomy and the creation of dependency start in the producer's loss of control over the nature, conditions, and product of his work—the expropriation of his work. Indeed, according to my postulate, the loss of autonomy of the citizen does not start in the sphere of consumption but in the world of production.

Bureaucratization of Work: A Product of Industrialization or of Class Control?

Another consequence of focusing on the world of consumption and not on the area of production and its class relations is that it leads Illich to misunderstand the nature of bureaucracy and bureaucratization of work in our societies. He just assumes that technological knowledge and the all-pervasive industrialization determine a division of labor that explains the appearance of production, trade, and services bureaucracies. But this explanation begs the questions of why that technological knowledge is distributed in the way that it is, and why that technology is frequently a vehicle of human oppression and not of liberation. Indeed, I would postulate that technology is not an independent force that fatalistically determines all relations, including social ones, but rather the reverse is true, i.e. the social relations (who controls what, and how this control takes place) determine the type of organization to be chosen and the type of technology to be used. As Braverman (38) has shown, (a) a historical review of "what preceded what" shows that the managerial revolution— Taylorism—and the bureaucratic form of organization that it created preceded the scientific revolution and not vice versa; and (b) that bureaucratic form of organization was and is created by the need of the employer—the manager—to structure and control the process of work. Indeed, that control is a major power of the employer. And characteristics of that structure and control are that (a) decision making has to be organized from the highest levels downwards, according to a vertical order of hierarchy in which the only ones who have complete control and a "complete picture" of the process of production are the controllers of that process; (b) technologies employed must not only enable, be compatible with, and replicate that hierarchical division of labor, but also fragment the nature of work, making every producer an expert of a small part—but not the whole—of the process; and (c) the distribution of technologies, skills, and knowledge must, within the constraints of (a) and (b), be compatible with the minimization of costs and the maximization of profits (39).

Within that process of production, technology and its requirements do not determine the hierarchical division of labor, but the hierarchical division of labor determines the type of technology used in that process. Technology, then, reinforces the already existing hierarchical and fragmentary division of labor. Indeed, that hierarchicalization is already there and is determined primarily by the class and sex roles existent in our societies. Let me illustrate this with an analysis of the responsibility that the members of the health team have. Within that health team, we find a well defined hierarchical order with the physician, most often a man of upper-middle-class extraction, at the top; below him, the supportive nurses, most often women with lower-middle-class backgrounds, and at the bottom, under both of them, we find the attendants and auxiliaries, the service workers, who most frequently are women of working-class backgrounds.[5] According to Illich and other industrialist theorists, what primarily explains that hierarchy are the different degrees of control over the technological knowledge necessary for the provision of industrialized medicine. But past and present experience shows that (a) the responsibilities that the different members of the team have are primarily due to their class backgrounds and sex roles, and only secondarily, very secondarily indeed, to their technological knowledge;[6] and (b) this technological knowledge, far from causing that cleavage and hierarchy among these members, merely reinforces that hierarchy. In that respect the acquisition of that knowledge—education and training—is the mere legitimation of that class and sex hierarchical distribution of power and responsibilities (40). Indeed, although the degree of technological knowledge developed in medicine has changed dramatically since the Flexner Report of 1910 to

[5]In this categorization, working class includes blue-collar, service, and farm workers. For a class analysis of the labor force in the health sector, see reference 40.

[6]Actually, due to the rapid rate of obsolescence of the technological knowledge in medicine, it is not infrequent to find knowledge to be more dysfunctional than functional.

the present, the class composition of the members of the health team has not changed significantly from that time.[7] Actually, the Flexnerian "revolution" in medicine and the creation of scientific medicine further strengthened but did not create that class distribution of responsibilities within the health sector that already existed. Indeed, to assume, as Illich does, that the distribution of responsibilities in medicine is due to its industrialization is to confuse symptoms with causes. It is *primarily* the class structure and the class relations of our society that determine that distribution. And, one could further postulate that this class structure and hierarchy militate against the provision of comprehensive medical care. For example, while most of the needs of the patients in our populations are those of care, most of the strategies within the health team and the health sector are directed by the "expert" in cure, the physician. The strategy for care within that team, however, would require (a) not the authoritarian (vertical), but the collaborative (horizontal) distribution of responsibilities, and (b) not a change from experts in cure to experts in care, but rather giving the team—including *all* its members as well as the patient—responsibility for both care and cure. However, the joint provision of the care, by the patient himself, his family, and all members of the team, is seriously handicapped in our class-structured society, where roles and functions are not distributed according to the need for them, but primarily according to the hierarchical order prevalent in our society, dictated by its class structure and class relations.

Structural Iatrogenesis: Industrialism or Capitalism?

Illich, by dismissing from the very beginning the categories of capitalism, class structure, and class relations, is seriously limited in finding the causes of his structural iatrogenesis. Indeed, while he attributes clinical iatrogenesis to the physicians, and social iatrogenesis to the medical care system, he finds structural iatrogenesis to be due to the culture of industrialization. Structural iatrogenesis, Illich writes, "is spawned by a cancerous delusion about life, and manifests itself when this delusion has pervaded a culture" (4, p. 160). And the creation of that culture that pervades "medical industry and civilization" is the symptom of the overall and pervasive process of industrialization. His solution for that iatrogenesis includes (a) reversing industrialization and its growth rate,

[7]Let me clarify in this footnote that I do believe there have been profound changes in the structure and composition of the labor force, including the labor force in the health sector. But most of these changes have taken place within each social class, not among social classes. For a further elaboration of this point, see reference 40.

(b) breaking down industrial bureaucracies, starting with the medical one, and (c) returning to self-reliance and enlightened self-interest. And in this struggle against industrialization and bureaucratization it is of paramount importance to start with medicine,

> since medicine is a sacred cow, its slaughter would have a "vibration effect": people who can face suffering and death without need for magicians and mystagogues are free to rebel against other forms of expropriation now practiced by teachers, engineers, lawyers, priests and party officials (4, p. 161).

But, by focusing on the medical bureaucracy as the "enemy," Illich misses the point because those bureaucracies are the servant of a higher category of power that I would define as the dominant class. Indeed, the empirical analysis of the health industry shows that contrary to what Illich believes, that industry is administered but not controlled by the medical profession. The analysis of power in the health sector in most Western developed societies shows that that power is primarily one of class, not of professional control. Indeed, those who have the first and final voice in the most important "corridors of power" in the health sector are the same corporate groups (composed mainly of the upper, corporate, or capitalist class) that control and/or have dominant influence in the organs—Illich's bureaucracies—of production, consumption, and legitimation in our societies. Indeed, as I have shown elsewhere,[8] members of the corporate class (owners and managers of financial capital), the class that has a dominant influence in the most important sphere of the U.S. economy—the monopolistic sector—have a dominant influence as well in the funding and reproductive institutions of the health industry (commercial insurance agencies, foundations, and teaching institutions). And members of the upper-middle class (executive and corporate representatives of middle-size enterprises and professionals, primarily corporate lawyers and financiers) have dominant influence in the delivery institutions. A similar situation appears with the executive and legislative branches of federal government that oversee and regulate the activities in the health sector. And in all these top agencies of power, the medical profession is represented only to a small degree. Indeed, the medical bureaucracy administers but does not control the health sector. And its power is delegated to it from the corporate and the upper-middle classes. Those classes and the medical profession share similar but not identical

[8]For a detailed presentation of the available evidence on the social class composition of the decision-making bodies in the U.S. health sector, see reference 40.

corporate and class interests, and if a conflict appears—and, as I postulate elsewhere (40), such conflict is bound to appear—then, it is quite clear who has dominant control in that situation, the same ones who have had that control from the *very beginning,* the corporate or dominant class. Indeed, one has to remember that the supporters and sponsors of "Flexnerian scientific medicine" were the Rockefeller and Carnegie Foundations, the voices of the corporate class of that period.

We find then that the main conflict in the health sector replicates the conflict in the overall social system. And that conflict is primarily not between the providers and consumers, but between those that have a dominant influence in the health system (the corporate class and upper-middle class) who represent less than 20 per cent of our population and control most of the health institutions, and the majority of our population (lower-middle class and working class) who represent 80 per cent of our population and who have no control whatsoever over either the production or the consumption of those health services (40). To focus then, as Illich and the majority of social critics do, on the conflict between consumers and medical providers as the most important conflict in the health sector, is to focus on a very limited and small part of the actual class conflict.

Actually, Illich's dismissal of the concept of social class as an irrelevant category for his analysis leads him to see the conflict in a compartmentalized way, i.e. as taking place among individual holders of skills and trades on the one hand, and the supposed benefactors of those skills and trades, the consumers, on the other. Thus he sees the "campagne dé bataille" in the control and redefinition of those skills and trades. But here again the conflict seen in this way begs the questions of (a) why those skills and roles are distributed in the way they are to begin with; and (b) why those skills and roles are very frequently vehicles more of oppression than liberation.

Regarding the first, the distribution of skills and roles in the medical sector, Illich assumes that what gives power to the medical profession is the exclusive control of those skills and trades, thus his suggestion of deprofessionalization. My answer however, is, as I have indicated, that those skills and trades reinforce and legitimate the power that is *already* there. The deprofessionalization of medicine and the dehierarchicalization of medicine, i.e. its democratization, are not possible within our class-structured society. The change of the latter is a prerequisite for the change of the former. The reverse, as Illich suggests, is unhistorical.

As to the frequently oppressive role of the medical bureaucracies,

Illich considers that they fail and determine oppression because they generate a self-serving addiction. His unawareness of social class structures and relations as the most important conceptual framework for understanding our institutional behavior, including the medical institutions, prevents him from understanding that services bureaucracies—including medicine—are, far from failing, succeeding in what they are supposed to do. Indeed, had Illich's analysis been historical and dialectical, he would have understood that the functions of the health industry are primarily determined outside and not inside the health sector. As Susser (41) has written, the concepts of health and of the types of health services have continuously changed and been redefined according to the needs of the capitalist mode and relations of production. And in this process of redefinition, the ones that have the dominant voice in defining health and health services have not been the medical bureaucracies as Illich writes, but the dominant class—the capitalist or corporate class. For example, when the economic needs (productivity of the system) and political needs (quieting social unrest) of that class so required in Britain, that class supported and passed the national health insurance of Lloyd George's government in 1911 in spite of the opposition of the medical profession (41). And today, as then, most of the changes in the definition of health and health services have occurred not because but in spite of the medical profession. A recent example has been the change of therapeutic practice in obstetrics with the provision of abortion on demand. That redefinition of health practice was due to the needs of the organs of legitimation—including the juridical organs—to respond to (a) an increasingly alienated and radicalized women's liberation movement, and (b) the population policies of the time.

In all these cases the redefinition of values, or what Galbraith (42) calls the convenient social virtues, followed the needs of the corporate class, not of the medical profession. Indeed, as Galbraith has recently indicated, the convenient social virtues are the ones that are primarily convenient to the most powerful in our society. Actually, what Galbraith and others are increasingly saying was said quite clearly by Marx (43):

> The ideas of the ruling class are in every *epoch* the ruling ideas: i.e. the class which is the ruling *material* force of society, is at the same time its ruling *intellectual* force. The class which has the means of material production at its disposal, has control at the same time over the means of mental production.

And health values and ideas are not an exception.

According to this explanation, then, the medical profession is a repository and guardian of the definition of those values, but not the ultimate definer. Reflecting the actual location of power, the profession has continuously lost its battle against that redefinition whenever its power had to be tested in a conflict with the corporate and dominant class.

In summary, and as I have shown elsewhere (40), one of the functions of the services bureaucracies—including the medical bureaucracy—is to legitimize and protect the system and its power relations. One aspect of that protection is social control—the channeling of dissatisfaction—which Illich introduces as structural iatrogenesis. But, to believe that social control is due to the culture of medicine and the pervasiveness of industrialization is to ignore the basic question of who regulates and most benefits from that control. An analysis of our societies shows that the services bureaucracies—including the medical ones—although willing accomplices in that control, are not the major benefactors. The ultimate benefactor of any social control intervention in any system is the dominant class in that system.

A Final Note on the Convergence Theory: The Possible Replication of Class Relations in Socialist Societies

As I have indicated, the main feature of the theory of convergence is that all societies, either capitalist or socialist, are converging toward similar social formations, i.e. industrialized societies. And these societies are held to be characterized by a similar process of industrialization that has determined the predominance of the bureaucracy as the primary social formation, with managers and technocrats having replaced the dominant classes in those societies. The supporters of that theory give the USSR and the Eastern European countries as examples of socialist societies which because of their high degree of industrial development also have full-fledged bureaucracies as the controllers of social and economic activity in each sector, and thus increasingly resemble our own Western industrialized societies.

This analysis, however, is too much of a simplification. Indeed, an analysis of the Eastern European societies, including the USSR, shows that the bureaucracies—including the medical bureaucracies—are not the primary controllers of each social and economic activity, but are subservient to a larger authority, the political party. Indeed, the planning, regulatory, and administrative responsibilities of the state bureaucracies are subject to the higher power of the upper echelons of the party. And these higher echelons of the party are the ones that have created the state bureaucracies, not vice versa. The power of the party is manifested and expressed through those bureaucracies. In this alternate explanation of bureaucratization of Eastern European societies, that bureaucratization was not the result of industrialization, but the result of the party's need to control the process of production and industrialization. And that party became a dominant class in itself when (a) it began to use its control over the means of production, not to optimize the producers' control over the process and means of production, but rather to optimize the production itself, i.e. when the accumulation of capital became the primary goal of those societies; and (b) it used its political control over the production, trade, and services bureaucracies not to decentralize and democratize them but to optimize its control by increasing the centralization and hierarchicalization of those bureaucracies.

As Sweezy has indicated, it was the belief of the political party in the 1920s, shared by both Stalinists and Trotskyists, that (a) democratization of the process of production was impossible in an underdeveloped society, and that (b) the need for capital accumulation had to be the first priority in the thirties and forties in preparing for and winning the Second World War. It was primarily these beliefs that led to the centralization of power that created bureaucratization and absence of institutional democratization. (For an extensive elaboration on this point, see the debate between Sweezy and Bettelheim presented in reference 44; see also Sweezy (45).) As Sweezy and Bettelheim have indicated, the appearance of a dominant class (the party), and its servants (the bureaucracies), determined the replication of class relations between dominant and dominated classes which were similar to, although not identical with, those in Western societies. In this process, the state bureaucracies were and are the administrative agencies of those relations, but did not generate those relations. Indeed, as Bettelheim (46, p. 46) says "there cannot exist a 'state power of the bureaucracy,' because a bureaucracy is always in the service of a dominant class."

In summary, in those Eastern European societies the bureaucracy is subject to and dependent on the political power of the party. And although there is considerable overlapping of membership among both, still, the bureaucrat and technocrat are both formally and informally dependent on the dominant class, the political party. The democratization of the former would require the democratization of the latter. Indeed, the struggle for institutional and industrial control that took place during the Cultural Revolution in China (which included a battle against elitism and bureaucratization in the medical sector) was part of a far wider and more important conflict, i.e. the conflict between large segments of the peasantry and the industrial working class and a sector of the political party that had ceased to be representative and had become instead an oppressive dominant force, a dominant class (46). Similarly in Cuba, the fight against bureaucratization in the middle sixties that Che Guevara stimulated was one component of a wider political conflict against a sector of the leadership of the Communist party—the Escalante group—that wanted to give priority to capital accumulation and to the efficiency of the system, over the democratization of the system (47).

And, in still another example, in Chile, the conflict in the health sector between large segments of the population and the majority of Chilean medical professionals, led by the Chilean Medical Association, was part of a far larger conflict over the socialization and democratization of the society. And the opposition of the medical profession to Allende was not because Allende reduced the amount of technology available to it, as Illich seems to believe, but because, in encouraging the democratization of the health institutions, he was a threat to the perpetuation of its social class as well as professional privileges. Indeed, when Illich (4, pp. 42–43) writes that

> by far the majority of Chilean doctors resisted the call of their President [to reduce the national pharmacopoeia]; many of the minority who tried to translate his ideas into practical programmes were murdered within one week after the take-over by the junta on September 11, 1973,

one has to realize that the savage assassination of the physicians and other health workers who supported Allende by the military junta (with the assistance of the majority of the Chilean medical profession), was an action far transcending the irritation over a reduction of technology. Illich's primary focus on technology, to the degree of making a fetish of it, seems to make him unaware of the fact that the fight in Chile was one, not primarily over technology, but over the class control of the health and all other institutions. Indeed, as I have indicated elsewhere (48), the majority of the medical profession in Chile reacted as much, if not more, against the curtailment of their class as of their professional privileges.

Actually, the experience in the socialist societies does not show, in my opinion, that capitalism and socialism converge, but that (a) the socialization of the means of production is a necessary but not sufficient condition for its democratization; (b) the class structure and class relations may reappear and be perpetuated in socialist societies, not because of industrialization, but because of the political centralization of power; (c) the conflict and struggle against bureaucratization and for democratic institutional control that occurred in China, Cuba, and Chile were part of a far larger and more important one, i.e. the struggle for the disappearance of class structures and for the political and economic democratization of those societies; and (d) to the degree that class control of the health institutions changed, the product and nature of those institutions changed. Indeed, even the definition and meaning of health changed from one where health was seen as an individual effort motivated by enlightened self-interest, to one of community and collective effort.

Final Comments on the Political Relevance of Illich

The Industrialization of Fetishism or the Fetishism of Industrialization

Having made a critique and review of Illich's writings, with primary focus on the area of health, and having postulated alternatives to both his explanations and his solutions, allow me to finish with some random thoughts about the political nature and relevancy of his two main suggestions for change: the reversal of industrialization, and the importance of self-reliance. In other words, a final note on the political uses and misuses of Illich's main messages.

As to the reversal of industrialization, I find Illich's emphasis on the process of industrialization as the culprit of his pains (iatrogeneses) quite a limiting one. Actually, by considering the industrialization and bureaucratization of our societies as the cause and not the symptom of our distribution of economic and political power, Illich seems to reduce all our political problems to managerial ones. In this way, he who resents the industrialization of all fetishism—including medicine—ends by fetishizing the process of industrialization itself. This fetishization of that process appears, for example, in his analysis of the most important public health problem in the world today: undernutrition. Here, once again, Illich assumes that industrialization is the major cause of the problem.

> Beyond a certain level of capital investment in the growing and processing of food, malnutrition must become pervasive . . . [and] what is happening in the sub-Saharan Sahel is only a dress rehearsal for the encroaching world famine. This is but the application of a general law. When more than a certain proportion of value is produced by the industrial mode, subsistence activities are paralysed, equity declines and the total satisfaction in that

particular area diminishes. In other words, beyond a certain level of industrial hubris, Nemesis *must* set in (4, pp. 155–156).

Absent in this analysis is the consideration of the critical political factors of who controls those economies (land and capital) and the process of industrialization. By focusing on the process of industrialization per se, and avoiding the economic and political conditions that determine underdevelopment and the type of industrialization that is used (the inter- and intra-country conditions of economic exploitation, the control of international trade, and other factors), his analysis seems aseptic and almost neutral. But, an alternative explanation to that of Illich's for underdevelopment and malnutrition is that certain types of industrialization (e.g. the Green Revolution) ostensibly exported from capitalist countries have reinforced and capitalized upon, but not generated, the already existing maldistribution of economic and political power, both within and among nations, the actual causes of their underdevelopment. Actually, Cuba and China, two of the very few countries in the sphere of underdevelopment that have controlled and almost solved their malnutrition problem, had to break with that maldistribution of power to allow them to use industrialization differently, not for the benefit of the few, but for the benefit of the many. The real problem the progressive forces in those countries faced in solving their malnutrition problem was not the process of centralized industrialization, but the centralization of economic and political power in the dominant oligarchies, allied with the corporate transnational interests, which determined that centralized industrialization. To change the latter they had to break with the former. Actually, the priest Camilo Torres in Columbia, who was assassinated while trying to change those economic and political structures, understood the causes of underdevelopment and malnutrition in Latin America far better than the urbane, sophisticated Ivan Illich in Mexico.

Indeed, the experiences in both China and Cuba would seem to indicate that the type of industrialization that exists in developing countries is a symptom but not a cause of their problems. (For an elaboration of this point, see reference 11.) In spite of these realities, endless interpretations of the political phenomena of underdevelopment are being advanced and sold, either under the pretense of the "population problem," or more recently, of the "problem of industrialization," that do not clarify but further obfuscate the actual economic and political causes of underdevelopment, whose reality and existence are increasingly clear for all to see.

The Limitations of Doing One's Own Thing

We are left then with Illich's second major suggestion for solving our problems: the self-reliance, self-care, independence, and autonomy of the individual citizen. But what is the meaning of this self-care? This aspect of Illich's strategy for change appears to me to be close, if not identical, to the strategy of that segment of American youth that joined in the "Woodstock nation," a strategy that basically relies on "life-style" solutions. And in that strategy, "doing one's own thing," or in Abbie Hoffman's words, "whatever the fuck we want" (quoted in 49), is not only the goal, but also the means for change, i.e. freedom and liberty defined as the lack of social constraints.

I postulate that the popularity of this strategy in our U.S. social environment and its appeal to the organs of legitimation—primarily the media—is because, rather than weakening, it strengthens the basic ethical tenets of bourgeois individualism, the ethical construct of capitalism where one has to be free to do whatever one wants, free to buy and sell, to accumulate wealth or to live in poverty, to work or not, to be healthy or to be sick. Far from being a threat to the power structure, this life-style politics complements and is easily co-optable by the controllers of the system, and it leaves the economic and political structures of our society unchanged. Moreover, the life-style approach to politics serves to channel out of existence any conflicting tendencies against those structures that may arise in our society.

Similarly, we find this life-style politics appearing increasingly in the health sector. Self-care and changes in life style are supposed to be the most important strategies to improve the health of our individual citizens. And behavioralists, psychologists, and "mood" analyzers are put to work to change the individual's behavior. In the words of one advocate of this approach:

> It is becoming increasingly evident that many health problems are related to individual behavior. In the absence of dramatic breakthroughs in medical science the greatest potential for improving health is through changes in what people do and do not do to and for themselves (50).

This strategy of self-care, however, assumes that the basic cause of his sickness or unhealth is the individual citizen himself, and not the system, and therefore the solution has to be primarily his and not the structural change of the economic and social system and its health sector. Not surprisingly, this emphasis on the behavior of the individual, not of the economic system, is welcomed and even exploited by those forces that benefit from the lack of change within the system. Interestingly, here in the health sector we again find the same analysis and strategies for change that we found in the sixties in the analysis of poverty in America. The sociological studies, for the most part, focused their analysis on the poor, not on the economic system that produced poverty. Thus, not paradoxically, most of the strategy for eradicating that poverty—the anti-poverty programs—was directed at the poor themselves, but not at the economic system that produced that poverty. Let me clarify that, today, we have even more poor people than we had before those programs started and the effect of those programs has been very limited indeed.

Similarly, in the health sector, a plethora of behavioral and sociological studies are devoted to analyzing the behavior of the individual, but very few studies exist that concern the behavior of the economic and political system that determines that behavior to start with. And most of the strategies for change are focused on changing the behavior of the individual and not the behavior of the system; thus, the appearance of self-care and health education strategies as possible and plausible strategies for change. But a far better strategy than self-care and changes in life style to improve the health of the individual, would be to change the economic and social structure that, according to my postulate, conditioned and determined that unhealthy individual behavior to start with. Let me give a specific example: the problem of the unhealthy diet of our citizens. The strategy of the life-style politics for correcting the unhealthy diet of our population, by individually changing the food consumption patterns (diet) of individual persons, avoids the political question of why the individuals consume that diet in the way they do. Thus, it ignores the enormous power of the economic needs of specific corporate interests in (a) determining that consumption, and (b) stimulating a certain type of production. Indeed, as Dr. Cornely (51), former president of the American Public Health Association, has indicated, a primary responsibility for the very poor diet of the U.S. citizens lies with the corporate practices of the food conglomerates. (For a presentation of the relationship between corporate practices of these main food corporations and the diet of children, see reference 51.) And these food conglomerates, as several studies have shown, are increasingly linked with the main sources of financial capital in this country, the most important sector of the corporate class and the one that has a dominant influence in most of the sectors of our economic system.

In the light of this iatrogenic economic and political environment, and the overwhelming power and influence of those economic groups, to speak of changes in life style as the proper strategy sounds to me to be not only very limited and unrealistic, but naive and sheer escapism. Indeed, I would postulate that unless the patterns of ownership and control of the means of production and consumption of the food and all other industries and sectors change in our society, from the control by the few to the control by the many, we will continue to have as poor a diet as we have today and have had in the past. And, thus, contrary to what Illich and others postulate, I believe that the greatest potential for improving the health of our citizens is not primarily through changes in the behavior of individuals, but primarily through changes in the patterns of control, structures, and behavior of our economic and political system. The latter could lead to the former. But the reverse is not possible.

Actually, it is precisely because of the impossibility of the reverse, and thus the lack of conflict between Illich's message and the basic tenets of our economic system, that his message, the life-style politics, is and increasingly will be presented by the organs of the media as the resolution of our crises and problems.

Indeed, Illich, radical in style but intrinsically conservative in message and substance, will be paraded as part of our solution. And at a time of increasing crises in our societies, the change in life styles, as opposed to political change, will be paraded as the solution. Indeed, I predict that powerful organs of value generation will be extremely sympathetic to Illich's emphasis on cultural as opposed to political change, stirring "new hopes in the hollow breast of at least one jaded revolutionary" (52). Cultural revolution will indeed be used to further postpone political change. And meanwhile, I postulate that to the same degree that the cultural politics of the Woodstock nation proved easily co-optable and irrelevant to the solutions of our problems in the sixties, this cultural revolution in our society will be similarly co-optable and equally irrelevant to the problems of our nation in the seventies. History will tell.

References

1. Cohen, N.M., and Backett, E.M. Medical nemesis. Book Review of *Medical Nemesis* by I. Illich. *Lancet* II (7895): 1503–1504, 1974.

2. Kozol, J. Quoted in I. Illich, *Deschooling Society*. Calder and Boyars, London, 1971.

3. Schwarzenberg, L. Le "bon sens" de Monsieur Illich. *Le Nouvel Observateur* 523: 3, 1974.

4. Illich, I. *Medical Nemesis: The Expropriation of Health.* Calder and Boyars, London, 1975.

5. Illich, I. Medical nemesis. *Lancet* I (7863): 918–921, 1974.

6. Illich, I. Medical nemesis: The destructive force of professional health care. *Social Policy* 5(2): 3–9, 1974.

7. Blackburn, R. A brief guide to bourgeois ideology. In *Student Power,* edited by A. Cockburn and R. Blackburn, pp. 163–213. Penguin Books, Baltimore, 1969.

8. Frankenberg, R. Functionalism and after? Theory and developments in social science applied to the health field. *Int. J. Health Serv.* 4(3): 411–427, 1974.

9. Galbraith, J.K. *The New Industrial State,* p. 389. Houghton-Mifflin, Boston, 1967.

10. Rostow, W.W. *The Stages of Economic Growth.* Cambridge University Press, Cambridge, 1962.

11. Navarro, V. The underdevelopment of health or the health of underdevelopment. *Int. J. Health Serv.* 4(1): 5–27, 1974. (Also included on pp. 3–32 of this volume.)

12. Kahn, H., and Wiener, A.J. *The Year 2,000.* Macmillan, New York, 1967.

13. Cronkite, W. Report on industrialization. CBS News, August 1973.

14. Bell, D. The post-industrial society: A speculative view. In *Scientific Progress and Human Values,* edited by E. Hutchings and E. Hutchings. American Elsevier, New York, 1967.

15. Aron, R. *Progress and Disillusion: The Dialectics of Modern Society.* Praeger, New York, 1968.

16. Illich, I. *Tools for Conviviality.* Calder and Boyars, London, 1971.

17. Illich, I. *Deschooling Society.* Calder and Boyars, London, 1971.

18. Friedman, M. *Capitalism and Freedom.* University of Chicago Press, Chicago, 1962.

19. Kessel, R.A. The A.M.A. and the supply of physicians. *Law and Contemporary Problems* 35: 267–283, 1970.

20. Kessel, R.A. Price discrimination in medicine. *Journal of Law and Economics* 1: 20–53, 1958.

21. Nixon, R.M. U.S. Presidential Address, 1972.

22. Navarro, V. From public health to health of the public: The redefinition of our task. *Am. J. Public Health* 64(6): 538–542, 1974.

23. Holland, W.W. Taking stock. *Lancet* II(7895): 1494–1497, 1974.

24. Haggerty, R.J. The boundaries of health care. *Pharos* 35(3): 106–111, 1972.

25. Miliband, R. *The State in Capitalist Society: An Analysis of the Western System of Power,* p. 10. Weidenfeld and Nicolson, London, 1969.

26. Schiller, H.I. *Mass Communications and American Empire.* Beacon, Boston, 1971.

27. Schiller, H.I. *The Mind Managers.* Beacon, Boston, 1974.

28. Servan Schreiber, J.L. *The Power to Inform.* McGraw-Hill, New York, 1974.

29. Marcuse, H. *One Dimensional Man.* Beacon, Boston, 1964.

30. Ollman, B. *Alienation.* Cambridge University Press, London, 1974.

31. Pappenheim, F. *The Alienation of Modern Man.* Monthly Review Press, New York, 1974.

32. Navarro, V. The underdevelopment of health of working America: causes, consequences, and possible solutions. *Am. J. Public Health* 66(6):538–547, 1976. (Also included on pp. 82–99 of this volume.)

33. Zernan, J. Organized labor versus "the revolt against work": The critical contest. *Telos* 21: 194–206, 1974.

34. Levison, A. *The Working Class Majority.* Coward, McCann, and Geoghegan, New York, 1974.

35. Dreitzel, H.P., editor. *The Social Organization of Health.* Macmillan, New York, 1971.

36. Howe, H.F. Health and work. Editorial. *Am. J. Public Health* 65(1): 82, 1975.

37. Special Task Force to the Secretary of Health, Education, and Welfare. *Work in America.* M.I.T. Press, Cambridge, Mass., 1973.

38. Braverman, H. *Labor and Monopoly Capital: The Degradation of Work in the Twentieth Century.* Monthly Review Press, New York and London, 1974.

39. Marglin, S.A. What do bosses do? The origins and functions of hierarchy in capitalist production. *The Review of Radical Political Economics* 6(2): 60–112, 1974.

40. Navarro, V. Social policy issues: An explanation of the composition, nature and functions of the present health sector of the United States. *Bulletin of the New York Academy of Medicine* 51(1) second series: 199–234, 1975. (Reprinted, in modified form, on pp. 135–169 of this volume.)

41. Susser, M. Ethical components in the definition of health. *Int. J. Health Serv.* 4(3): 539–548, 1974.

42. Galbraith, J.K. *Economics and the Public Purpose,* p. 31. Houghton-Mifflin, Boston, 1972.

43. Marx, K. The German ideology. In *Selected Works,* Vol. 1, p. 47. Lawrence and Wishart, London, 1962. (Quoted in C.H. Anderson, *The Political Economy of Social Class,* p. 60. Prentice-Hall, Englewood Cliffs, N.J., 1974.)

44. Sweezy, P., and Bettelheim, C. *On The Transition to Socialism.* Monthly Review Press, New York and London, 1971.

45. Sweezy, P. The nature of Soviet society. *Monthly Review* 26(6): 1–16, 1974.

46. Bettelheim, C. *Cultural Revolution and Industrial Organization in China: Changes in Management and the Division of Labor.* Monthly Review Press, New York and London, 1974.

47. Boorstein, E. *The Economic Transformation of Cuba.* Monthly Review Press, New York and London, 1968.

48. Navarro, V. What does Chile mean: An analysis of events in the health sector before, during and after Allende's administration. *Health and Society, Milbank Mem. Fund Q.* 52(2): 93–130, 1974. (Also included on pp. 33–66 of this volume.)

49. Silber, I. *The Cultural Revolution,* p. 58. Times Change Press, New York, 1970.

50. Fuchs, V. Health care and the United States economic system. *Milbank Mem. Fund Q.* 50(2, part 1): 211–237, 1972.

51. Cornely, P.B. The hidden enemies of health and the American Public Health Association. *Am. J. Public Health* 61(1): 7–18, 1971.

52. Toynbee, P. Quoted among press opinions of Illich's works, I. Illich, *Medical Nemesis,* p. 184. Calder and Boyars, London, 1975.

PART III:
THE POLITICAL ECONOMY
OF MEDICAL CARE

An Explanation of the Composition, Nature, and Functions of the Present Health Sector of the United States

By Way of Introduction

In trying to understand the present composition, nature, and functions of the health sector in the United States, one is hampered by a great scarcity of literature, both in the sociological and the medical care fields, that would explain how the shape and form of the health sector—the tree—is determined by the same economic and political forces shaping the political and economic system of the United States—the forest. In fact, health services literature reveals what C.W. Mills (1), Birnbaum (2), and others (3, 4) have found in other areas of social research: a predominance of empiricism, leading to dominance of experts on trees who neither analyze nor question the forest but accept it as given.

Health services research, like most social research, has become more and more compartmentalized, with its practitioners turning into narrower and narrower specialists, superbly trained in their own fields, but with less and less comprehension of the total. And yet, the Hegelian dictum that "the truth is the whole" continues with its undiminished validity. Let me underline that I am not belittling empirical studies, i.e. the analysis of detail. Actually, the reader will see that I borrow heavily from the findings of empirical studies. But, as Baran and Sweezy (5) have indicated, "just as the whole is always more than the sum of the parts, so the amassing of small truths about the various parts and aspects of society can never yield the big truths about the social order itself." There is, indeed, a need for explanation of how the parts are related to each other, and it is in meeting this need that our empiricists have fallen short and, for the most part, have remained silent. It is to break this deafening silence that this article has been written. Although admittedly full of assumptions, perceptions, and values, it will try to show that the composition and distribution of health resources are determined by the same forces that determine the distribution of economic and political power in our society. Indeed, I would postulate that the former cannot be understood without an understanding of the latter.

The article is divided into three sections. The first is an analysis of the current social class and economic structures of the United States, both outside and within the health sector. The second analyzes the different degrees by which social class influences and controls the financing and delivery of care in health institutions, and the third analyzes the effects of class on the organs of the state. It is theorized that these social class influences on the institutions of production, reproduction, and legitimization determine the composition, nature, and functions of the health sector.

The Class Structure of the United States, Outside and Within the Health Sector

In attempting to explain and understand the composition, functions, and nature of the health sector, one must look outside the health sector and first address a key question in any society, i.e. who owns and who controls the income and wealth of that society?[1] Thus, I have to revive a forgotten paradigm in social analysis in the United States: that of social class structure. In so doing, I am going against the mainstream of our sociological research, which assumes that this category has been transcended by the present reality of the United States, where it is considered that most of our population is middle class. Actually, it is assumed in most of the press and in most of academia that the contemporary United States, and the rest of the Western democracies for that matter, are being recast in a mold of middle-class conditions and styles of life.[2] Moreover, this situation is considered to be the result of social fluidity and mobility that are believed to falsify past characterizations of the United States as a class society. This conclusion, however, seems to confuse class consciousness with class interests. Indeed, the social reality that establishes the level of social aspiration of the American population as the consumption pattern of the middle class, and the assumed concomitant absence of class consciousness, do not deny the existence of social classes. In fact, as C.W. Mills (9) pointed out,

> . . . the fact that men are not "class conscious" at all times and in all places does not mean that "there are no classes" or that "in America everybody is

[1]Simply stated, income is money coming from different sources, either as wages and salaries, dividends and profits, or as rent. Wealth is the value of people's possessions and property.

[2]An example of a recent newspaper article exhibiting this belief is that by Kumpa (6). The most influential of the large body of sociological literature that negates the existence of classes in the United States is Bell (7). For a critique of this literature, see reference 8.

middle class." The economic and social facts are one thing. Psychological feelings may or may not be associated with them in rationally expected ways. Both are important, and if psychological feelings and political outlooks do not correspond to economic or occupational class, we must try to find out why, rather than throw out the economic baby with the psychological bath, and so fail to understand how either fits into the national tub.

Actually, there is not even convincing evidence that class consciousness or awareness do not exist. According to a study conducted in 1964, 56 per cent of all Americans said that they thought of themselves as "working class," some 39 per cent considered themselves "middle class," and 1 per cent said they were "upper class." Only 2 per cent rejected the whole idea of class (10).

An analysis of the social structure of the United States shows that there are indeed social classes in this country. Since I have detailed this class structure elsewhere in this volume,[3] I will only summarize it here. In such an analysis, we find at the top of our society the upper or corporate class which, by virtue of its ownership of a disproportionate share of the personal wealth and/or its control over that wealth, commands the most important sectors of our society. At the other extreme of the social spectrum, we find the working class, composed primarily of industrial or blue-collar workers as well as farm workers and workers in the services sector. In between these two polar classes, there is the middle class, divided into upper and lower groupings and comprised of (a) professionals, (b) the business middle-class, (c) self-employed shopkeepers and craftsmen, and (d) office and sales workers. While aware of the simplifications that such a categorization implies, for reasons of brevity I shall refer to groups (a) and (b) as the upper-middle class, and groups (c) and (d) as the lower-middle class.

And the distribution of wealth and income closely follow these class lines, with the highest possession of both at the top and the lowest possession at the bottom, with a large gap in between. Using one of his excellent graphic analogies, Samuelson makes this skewed distribution quite clear. He states, in the eighth edition of *Economics,* "If we made today an income pyramid out of a child's blocks, with each layer portraying $1,000 of income, the peak would be far higher than the Eiffel

---

[3]See "The Underdevelopment of Health of Working America: Causes, Consequences and Possible Solutions," included in this volume, especially Figure 1 which sets forth the occupational and social class distribution in the U.S. and gives the annual median income for each category.

Tower, but almost all of us would be within a yard of the ground (11, p. 110). Moreover, these distribution patterns of wealth and income have remained remarkably constant over time. In the last retrospective study of the distribution of income, published in the 1974 annual *Economic Report of the President* (12) and widely reported in the press, it was found that "the bottom 20 per cent of all families had 5.1 per cent of the nation's income in 1947 and had almost the same amount (5.4 per cent) in 1972. At the top, there was a similar absence of significant change. The richest 20 per cent had 43.3 per cent of the income in 1947 and 41.4 per cent in 1972" (13).

This class structure in our society is also reflected in the composition of the different elements that participate in the health sector, either as owners, controllers, or producers of services. Indeed, considering just the health sector, and analyzing the owners, controllers, and producers of services in health institutions, we find that members of the upper class and, to a lesser degree, the upper-middle class (groups a and b of the middle class in the previous categorization), predominate in the decision-making bodies of our health institutions, i.e. the boards of trustees of foundations, teaching hospital institutions, medical schools, and hospitals. For the producers and the members of the labor force in the health sector we can see the distribution shown in Figure 1. At the top we find the physicians, who are mainly of upper-middle-class backgrounds and who had in 1970 a median annual net income of $40,000, which places them in the top 5 per cent of our society. I should add that the majority of persons in this group are white and male, besides being upper-middle class. They represent 7.3 per cent of the whole labor force in the health sector.

Below, very much below the upper class of the health sector, we find the level called paraprofessional. This could be defined as equivalent to the lower-middle-class category of office worker of the previous categorization (group d), i.e. nurses, therapists, technologists, and technicians, whose annual median income was approximately $6,000 in 1970. They represent 28.5 per cent of the labor force in the health sector. This group is primarily female and is part of the lower-income group. Nine per cent is black.

Below this group we find the working class per se of the health sector, the auxiliary, ancillary, and service personnel, representing 54.2 per cent of the labor force, who are predominantly women (84.1 per cent) and who include an overrepresentation of blacks (30 per cent). This group's median income was $4,000 in 1970.

Figure 1

Persons employed in the delivery of health services in the United States, by sex, in 1970

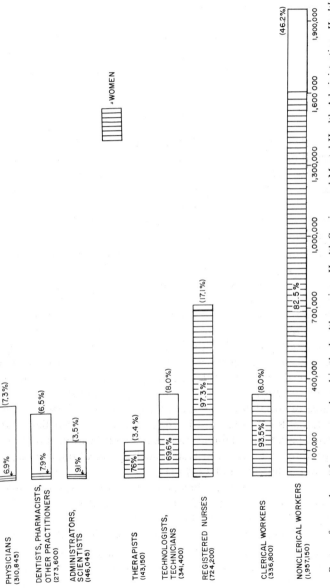

Source: for numbers of persons employed in the health services, Health Services and Mental Health Administration, *Health Resources Statistics: Health Manpower and Health Facilities, 1971,* U.S. Government Printing Office, Washington, D.C., 1972. Source for percentage of women physicians, M.Y. Pennell and J.E. Renshaw, Distribution of women physicians, 1970, *Journal of the American Medical Women's Association* 27(4): 197–203, 1972. Source for other categories, U.S. Bureau of the Census, 1970.

If we look at income distribution in the health sector, as we did for society in general, we find a similar structure, although here again, we find a great scarcity of information and a great absence of empirical data. Figure 2, however, shows the trend in the differentials of median income among the different groups of producers in the health sector from 1949 to 1970. Here we can see that there has been a very dramatic increase in the income differential between the top and bottom income groups of the health industry.

The Determinants of Income Differentials

Much has been written about the reasons for these income differentials. According to the orthodox economic paradigm, "every agent of production receives the amount of wealth that agent creates" and "every man receives all that he creates." Thus, workers' incomes depend on their productivity, i.e. "on the amount of capital available, on the one hand, and on workers' skills and education, on the other."[4] According to this interpretation, the conditions for social mobility are (a) increased education, to improve the workers' position in the market for their skills, and (b) equal opportunity for each worker in the competitive labor market. The strategy, then, is to increase educational opportunities and to break with the race and sex discrimination which prevents the proper functioning of the market forces. This paradigm is shared, incidentally, by the majority of people in the black and women's liberation movements within and outside the health sector. However, absent in this analysis is the concept of property and class. Actually, one of the widely accepted theoretical works on social inequality in today's United States, Rawls' *A Theory of Justice* (15), does not even mention the value of property as a source of social cleavage. Indeed, following the Weberian interpretation of status, Rawls and most of the exponents of what Barry (16) calls the liberal paradigm, maintain that social stratification is multidimensional, depending on a variety of factors such as education, income, occupation, religion, ethnicity, and so on (17).

Empirical evidence, however, seems to question the main assumptions of the liberal paradigm. Regarding the social mobility that is supposed to be the result of the widening of opportunities and of the free flow of labor market forces, and that is supposed to have caused the

[4]All these quotations are from Clark (14), the first work to enunciate the marginal productivity of income distribution. The most important contemporary work in this area is Samuelson (11).

Figure 2

The rise in income of selected personnel in the delivery of health services
in the United States, 1949–1970

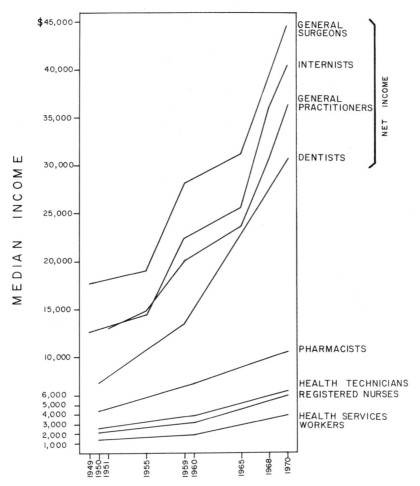

Source: for income of physicians, Continuing Survey of Physicians, Medical Economics
Company, Oradell, N.J., 1972. Figures are for self-employed physicians in solo practice,
under age 65. Source for income of dentists, Continuing Survey of Dentists, *Journal of the
American Dental Association,* various years. Source for income of other wage groups, U.S.
Bureau of the Census, *Statistical Abstract of the United States,* U.S. Government Printing
Office, Washington, D.C. 1950, 1960, and 1970.

withering away of the social classes, Westergaard (18) and others have recently shown that although there has been some mobility among the different social groups or strata within each social class, there has been practically no mobility among social classes.

And the primary objective of education, instead of being the transmission of skills to aid upward mobility, seems to have been the perpetuation of social roles within the predefined social classes. Indeed, Bowles and Gintis (19), among others, have indicated how education, labor markets, and industrial structures interact to produce distinctive social strata *within* each class. A similar situation prevails in the health sector, where Simpson (20) and Robson (21) in England, and Kleinbach (22) in the United States have shown how (a) the social class background of the main groups within the health labor force has not changed during the last 25 years, and how (b) education fixes and perpetuates those social backgrounds and replicates social roles. Actually, let me point out here that Flexner himself saw that as a function of medical education when he wrote that a primary aim of medical education was to separate the gentlemen (the upper class) from the quacks (the lower class).

Education, as a perpetuation of social roles, remains the same today as in Flexner's time. Simpson (20, p. 39), for instance, mentions that, within the five-scale grouping of classes in Britain, the offspring of social classes 1 and 2 (equivalent to our upper and upper-middle classes, as defined before) predominate in medicine:

> In 1961 more than a third were from class 2, rather less than a third from class 3, and only 3 per cent from classes 4 and 5 together. By 1966, social class 1 was contributing nearly 40 per cent. The proportion of children of classes 1 and 2 in universities generally, derived from the Robbins Report, is about 59 per cent. Individual medical schools vary between 69 and 73 per cent. It is hard to believe that the small number of medical students selected from families of low average income exhausts the potentially good students contained in this large part of the population.

That this situation may even follow a predefined policy is indicated in the following statement from the Royal College of Surgeons (23):

> . . . there has always been a nucleus in medical schools of students from cultured homes. . . . This nucleus has been responsible for the continued high social prestige of the profession as a whole and for the maintenance of medicine as a learned profession. Medicine would lose immeasurably if the proportion of such students in the future were to be reduced in favour of the precocious children who qualify for subsidies from the Local Authorities and State purely on examination results.

A similar situation occurs in the United States, where Lyden, Geiger, and Peterson (24) reported in 1968 that only 17 per cent of physicians were the children of craftsmen or skilled and unskilled laborers (who represented 57 per cent of the whole labor force), while over 31 per cent of physicians were children of professionals (representing 4.9 per cent of the labor force). Figure 3 depicts the recent changes in the race, sex and class composition of U.S. medical students. It is quite interesting and, I would add, not surprising, to note that while the underrepresentation of women and blacks among new entrants to the medical schools slowly, but steadily, diminished over the last decade, the underrepresentation of entrants with working-class and lower-middle-class backgrounds remained remarkably constant during the same period (25). Indeed, women, who represent 51 per cent of the U.S. population, made up 6 per cent of all medical students in 1961 and 17 per cent in 1973, while blacks, representing 12 per cent of the overall U.S. population, went during the same time period from 3 to 9 per cent of all medical students. During these years the percentage of medical students who came from families earning the median family income or below, representing approximately one-half of the population, remained at 12 per cent. This percentage, incidentally, has remained the same since 1920.

These accumulated bits of evidence would seem to indicate that there is not an automatic trend toward diminishing class differences or bringing about social class mobility within and outside the health sector of the present United States, and, I would postulate, in that of most Western European societies. As in the past, experience seems to show that, as Harold Laski used to say, "the careful selection of one's own parents" remains among the most important variables explaining one's own power, wealth, income, and opportunities. The importance of this selection, moreover, seems to be particularly vital at the top. As C.W. Mills (26) said, "It is very difficult to climb to the top . . . it is much easier and much safer to be born there."

It would seem, then, that the liberal paradigm does not sufficiently explain the composition of the labor force and its class and income structure. Indeed, I would postulate that a better explanation of that structure would be that the inequalities of income, wealth, and, as we will see in a later section, economic and political power, are functionally related to the way in which the means of production and reproduction of goods, commodities, and services, and the organs of legitimization in the United States, are owned, controlled, influenced, and directed. According to this interpretation, property and control of, and/or influence on, those means of production, reproduction, and legitimization are not just

Figure 3

Changes in the Race, Sex, and Class Composition of the
U.S. Population and of Medical Students

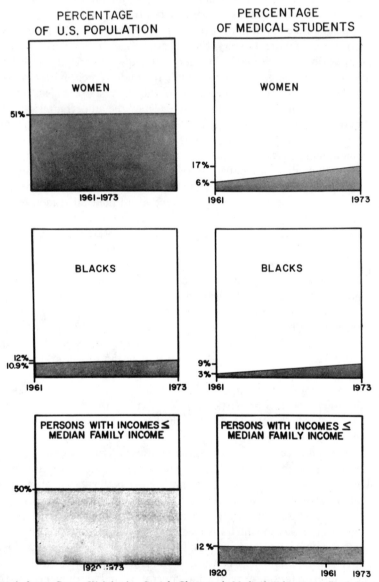

Adapted from Grace Kleinbach, *Social Class and Medical Education.* Cambridge,
Massachusetts, Department of Education, Harvard University (in preparation).

marginal factors in explaining class structure and income differentials, as the liberal paradigm would suggest, but key explanatory ones. Thus, in this alternative explanation, the overall distribution of wealth and income depends on who owns, controls, influences, and directs the means of production, reproduction, and legitimization in the different sectors of the U.S. economy. Overall income differentials among social classes, then, do not have so much to do with the free operation of the labor market forces, but more with the patterns of ownership and control of the main means of income-producing wealth and of the organs of legitimization, i.e. communication, education, and the agencies of the state. And according to this alternate explanation, education and other means of socialization are not the means of creating upward mobility among social classes, but actually are means of perpetuating patterns of control and ownership.

In summary, it can be postulated that social classes and income differentials come about because of the different degrees of ownership, control, and influence that different social classes have over the means of production and consumption and over the organs of legitimization, including the media, communications, education, and even the organs of state. Moreover, it can further be postulated that, as I will try to show in the following sections, these class influences determine not only the nature of the economic sectors in the United States today but also of the social sectors, including that of the health services. But, before discussing this, allow me to briefly outline the different sectors of our economy and their class composition, as a necessary prologue to explaining the nature, role, and functions of the health sector.

The Monopolistic, Competitive, and State Sectors of the U.S. Economy

O'Connor (27) and Galbraith (28), among others, have recently defined three different sectors in the United States economy: the planned or monopolistic sector, the market or competitive sector, and the state sector.

The first, the *planned or monopolistic sector,* which roughly employs a third of the labor force, is characterized by being capital- as opposed to labor-intensive, national in contrast to regional or local, and highly monopolistic both in economic concentration and in economic behavior (e.g. in the use of price fixing). Important characteristics of this sector are its requirements for economic stability and planning and a tendency toward vertical integration (e.g. the control of raw materials from the point of extraction to the process of production and distribution) as well as horizontal integration (i.e. the control of different vertical sectors of the industry and the establishment of conglomerates). If we look at the social makeup of this sector, we find (a) the corporation owners (the stock-holders) and the controllers (or managers), who Galbraith (28) says together make up the "corporate community" and whom Miliband (29) labels the "large business community," and whom, according to my own definition outlined before, we would call the corporate class; (b) the technocracy or professionals; (c) the blue-collar workers, highly union-ized in this sector, who correspond to the industrial working class of my previous categorization; and (d) the white-collar workers, the technical and administrative workers, or lower-middle class.

The second sector, the *market or competitive sector,* used to be the largest of the three sectors but today is the smallest and continues to decline. It employs roughly less than one-third of our labor force, with the largest proportion of workers being in services and distribution (27). It is characterized by being labor-intensive, local or regional in scope, with a relatively weak labor force and low unionization. Examples of workers in this sector are people working in restaurants, drug stores, commercial display, etc. The social makeup of this sector consists of (a) the owners and controllers (executives) of small-scale, localized industries and services, (b) small percentages of blue-collar workers and (c) of white-collar workers, and (d) a large sector of service workers, who are primarily auxiliary and ancillary personnel.

The third major sector is the *state sector,* which is made up of two subsectors. The first subsector produces goods and services under the direction of the state itself, e.g. the public health services, and the second involves production organized by industries under contract from the state. The contracts, e.g. for military equipment and supplies, are mainly with corporations belonging to the monopolistic sector. In terms of social makeup, the first subsector, employing close to 17 per cent of the labor force, has characteristics similar to those of the market system, while the other—the contractual one—also employs 17 per cent of the labor force and is part of the monopolistic sector. Figure 4 summarizes the percentage of the labor force in each sector and Figure 5 the main characteristics of the production and labor force in each sector.

Of these three sectors, the most important one for an explanation of the present economic system of the United States and also, according to my postulate, for a partial explanation of the situation in the health field, is the monopolistic sector. Actually, the owners and controllers of that sector, the American corporate class, have a pervasive and constantly felt

Figure 4
Approximate percentage of labor force in each sector
of the U.S. economy

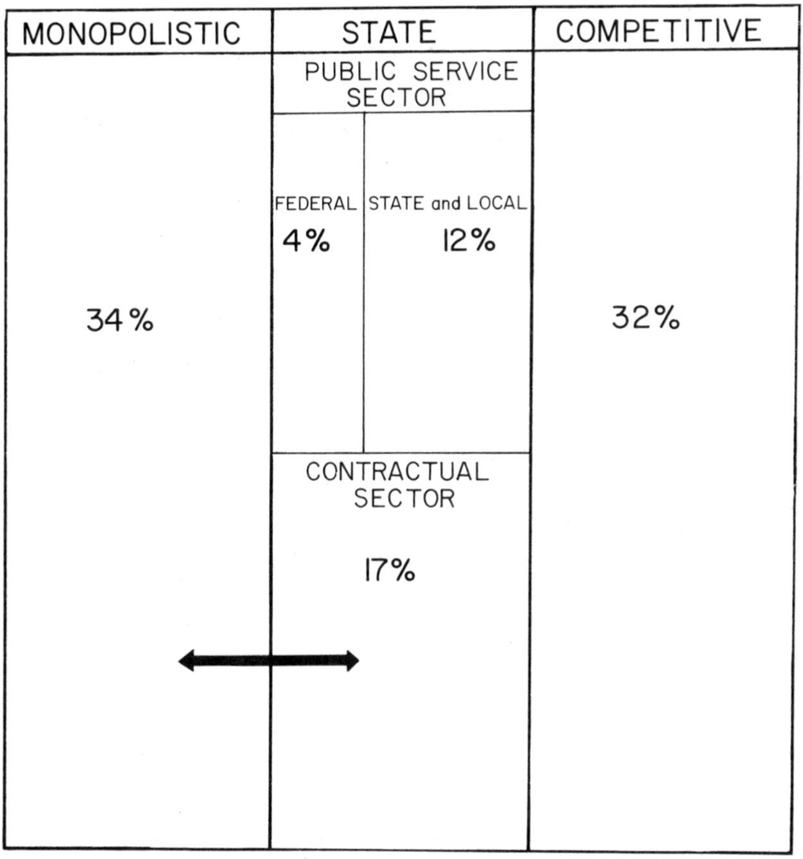

MONOPOLISTIC	STATE			COMPETITIVE
	PUBLIC SERVICE SECTOR			
	FEDERAL 4%	STATE and LOCAL 12%		
34%				32%
	CONTRACTUAL SECTOR 17%			
	←——————→			

Sources: references 27 and 30.

dominant influence over the patterns of production and consumption of the United States.[5] Their influence affects the most important means of

[5] By dominant or hegemonic influence I mean that influence which is most important in determining "an order in which a certain way of life and thought is dominant, in which one concept of reality is diffused throughout society in all its institutional and private manifestations, informing with its spirit all taste, morality, customs, religious and political principles, and social relations, particularly in their intellectual and moral connotations" (31).

Figure 5
Production and labor force characteristics of each sector
of the U.S. economy

	MONOPOLISTIC	STATE		COMPETITIVE
		CONTRACTUAL	SERVICE	
CHARACTERISTICS OF PRODUCTION	• PRIMARILY MANUFACTURING		• PRIMARILY SERVICE	• PRIMARILY TRADE and SERVICE
	• ECONOMIC CONCENTRATION		• ECONOMIC DECONCENTRATION	• ECONOMIC DECONCENTRATION
	• HIGHLY MONOPOLISTIC		• MONOPOLISTIC	• COMPETITIVE
	• VERTICAL and HORIZONTAL INTEGRATION (CONGLOMERATES)		• VERTICAL and SECTORIAL	• VERTICAL and SECTORIAL
	• NATIONAL and INTERNATIONAL		• FEDERAL, STATE, LOCAL	• REGIONAL and LOCAL
CHARACTERISTICS OF LABOR FORCE	• PREDOMINANTLY MALE		• PREDOMINANTLY FEMALE	• PREDOMINANTLY FEMALE
	• NONWHITES: UNDERREPRESENTED		• NONWHITES: PROPORTIONALLY REPRESENTED	• NONWHITES: OVERREPRESENTED
	• UNIONIZED		• NONUNIONIZED	• NONUNIONIZED
	• SALARIES: RELATIVELY HIGH		• SALARIES: MEDIUM	• SALARIES: LOW

production and distribution in the United States, as well as the means of
value generation, including the media and the educational institutions,
and the organs of the state.

I believe that in the health sector, that same class, augmented in this
case by the upper middle classes (the professionals and the business
middle class of my categorization), maintains a dominant influence on (a)
the financial and health delivery institutions, (b) the health teaching
institutions, and (c) the organs of the state in the health sector.[6]

The Control of the Financial and Health Delivery Institutions

The Structure of the Monopolistic Sector and Its Meaning in the Health Sector of the United States

A main characteristic of the economies of the United States and most
western nations is the high concentration of economic wealth in the
monopolistic sector. Table 1, for instance, shows the extremely high
concentration of corporate assets in comparatively few firms. In 1967, at
the top a few giant corporations (958, or just 0.06 per cent) held a
majority of all assets ($1,070 billion, or 53.2 per cent), while at the
bottom, a large number of small corporations (906,458, or 59 per cent of
the total) held a very small, almost minuscule portion of corporate assets
($31 billion, or 1.5 per cent).

[6]In this article I will limit myself to an analysis of the influence of the corporate classes and
upper-middle classes on the federal executive and legislative.

Table 1

Distribution of corporate assets for all U.S. corporations in 1967[a]

Minimum Assets	Corporations	Assets Owned
$	%	%
0	59.00	1
100,000	29.00	5
500,000	10.00	10
5,000,000	1.94	31
250,000,000	0.06	53
Total	100.00	100

[a] Source, data from U.S. Internal Revenue Service: Statistics of Income, *Corporation Income Tax Returns*. U.S. Government Printing Office, Washington, D. C., 1967.

This concentration of corporate economic power replicates itself in the several sectors that constitute the United States economy. For example, in the key sector of manufacturing, in 1962 a mere 100 firms (out of a total of 180,000 corporations and 240,000 unincorporated businesses) owned 58 per cent of the net capital assets of all the hundreds of thousands of manufacturing corporations. Another way of expressing this extraordinary degree of concentration is that, as Hunt and Sherman (32, p. 270) point out, "the largest 20 manufacturing firms owned a larger share of the assets than the smallest 419,000 firms combined."[7]

Another sector within the corporate side of the economy is the financial capital sector, which includes the banks, trusts, and insurance companies. Highly concentrated itself (according to the Pattman report (34) the 100 largest banks—out of a total of 13,775 commercial banks— hold 45 per cent of all deposits), this group exerts a dominant influence in the corporate sector, primarily through lending to the corporations. Actually, as a Congressional Committee report (33) indicated recently, accumulated evidence shows that corporations are not self-sufficient in terms of financial capital, but are increasingly dependent on the financial institutions for their capital needs. This dependency leads to influence on corporate policies by the financial capital institutions, through ownership of corporate stocks and the interlocking of directorships in their boards. As Morton Mintz (35) of the *Washington Post* wrote in summarizing the findings of that report, "Most of the nation's largest corporations appear

[7]There are several references showing the concentration of corporate wealth in this country. See the chapter "Monopoly Power: Increasing or Decreasing?" pp. 267–282, in Hunt and Sherman (32) and also reference 33.

to be dominated or controlled by eight institutions, including six banks." Through their boards, these banks have a close interlocking relationship with insurance companies such as Aetna Life, Prudential, and others. And it may give you an idea of the formidable concentration of power in those finance institutions when I tell you that, again according to that report, the top four banks in the country own 10 per cent of ITT stocks, 12 per cent of Xerox, 22 per cent of Gulf Oil, 10 per cent of International Paper, 12 per cent of Polaroid, and parts of many, many other powerful corporations. The importance of these figures may be shown by the fact that the House Banking and Currency Subcommittee of the U.S. Congress has stated that a 5 per cent ownership of stock in a corporation is sufficient to give the owners of the stock a controlling vote in that corporation (35).

Not surprisingly, the top financial institutions are also important in the health industry, the second largest industry in the country. According to the *National Journal* (36), the flow of health insurance money through private insurance companies in 1973 was $29 billion, slightly less than half of the total insurance—health and other—sold in this country in that year. About $15 billion, or over half of this money, flowed through the commercial insurance companies. Among these companies, we find, again, a high concentration of financial capital, with the ten largest commercial health insurers (Aetna, Travellers, Metropolitan Life, Prudential, CNA, Equitable, Mutual of Omaha, Connecticut General, John Hancock, and Provident) controlling close to 60 per cent of the entire commercial health insurance industry. Most of these top health insurance companies are also the biggest life insurance companies, which are, with the banks, the most important controllers of financial capital in this country. Metropolitan Life and Prudential, for instance, each control $30 billion in assets, making them far larger than General Motors, Standard Oil of New Jersey, and ITT (37). These financial entities have close links with banking, and through the banks they exercise a powerful influence over the top corporations. An example of this influence is that, out of 28 directors of Metropolitan Life, 23 also sit on the boards of banking institutions, particularly of the Chase Manhattan Bank (37), which owns 10 per cent of the stocks of American Airlines, 8 per cent of those of United Airlines, 15 per cent of the Columbia Broadcasting System, 6 per cent of Mobil Oil, and portions of very many other corporations (35). The importance of this influence, defined by some, such as the Subcommittee on Government Operations of the U.S. Senate, as dominance over the overall economy, is reflected in the present debate on the different proposals for national health insurance on whether to "open the doors" to the commercials or keep them out of the coming national health insurance scene. It actually speaks highly of the great political influence and power of these financial capital institutions that all the proposals, with the exception of the Kennedy-Griffith proposal whose main constituency was the trade unions of the monopolistic sector, i.e. AFL-CIO and UAW, have left room for, and even encouraged, the involvement of the commercials in the health sector. The Nixon, and now the Ford administration's proposal, for example, would increase the flow of money through the private insurance industry (including commercial health insurance) from \$29 to \$42 billion, with another \$14 billion handled by the private carriers in their role as intermediaries in the publicly financed segment of the proposed plan (36). Actually, it was the power of the commercial insurance companies that determined a change in the Kennedy-Griffith proposal—the only proposal which excluded the insurance companies—to one of acceptance of their role in the new Kennedy-Mills proposal. In fact, as a recent editorial in the *New York Times* (38) indicated, the decision of the Kennedy-Mills proposal "to retain the insurance companies' role was based on recognition of that industry's power to kill any legislation it considers unacceptable. The bill's sponsors thus had to choose between appeasing the insurance industry and obtaining no national health insurance at all."

We can see, then, how the same financial and corporate forces that are dominant in shaping the American economy also increasingly shape the health services sector. The commercial insurance companies, however, although the largest financial power in the premium market in the health sector, are not the only ones. They compete with the power of the providers, expressed in the insurance sector primarily through the Blues—Blue Cross and Blue Shield. The controllers of both the commercials and the Blues, although sharing class interests, have opposite and conflicting corporate interests. Actually, it is likely that the predominance of financial capital in the health sector, and specifically of commercial insurance, could mean the weakening of the providers' control of the health sector, analogous to the way in which the predominance of the monopolistic sector—financial and corporate—has meant the weakening of the market or competitive sector. If this should come about, we would probably see the proletarianization of the providers, with providers being mere employees of the finance corporations—the commerical insurance companies. In this respect, unionization of the medical profession would be a symptom of its proletarianization, so that the present incipient but steady trend toward unionization of the medical profession may be an indication of things to come in the health sector (39).

The Control of the Health Institutions: The Reproductory Ones

In order to understand the patterns of control and/or influence in the health sector, we have to look not only at the patterns of control in the financing of health services, but also at the patterns of control and influence in the health delivery institutions. Indeed, financial capital—the money or energy that moves the system—goes through prefixed institutional channels that are owned, controlled, and/or influenced by classes and groups which are similar to, although not identical with, those who have dominant influence through financing. We can group the institutions into (a) those that have to do with the reproduction and legitimization of the patterns of control and influence, e.g. the teaching institutions, and (b) those that deliver the services themselves. Indeed, following this categorization, we could speak of reproductive versus distributive institutions.

The former, in which I would include the foundations (e.g. the Johnson, Rockefeller, and Carnegie Foundations) besides the teaching medical institutions, are controlled by the financial and corporate communities and by the professionals, i.e. the corporate class and the upper-middle class of my initial categorization. As Professor MacIver (40) writes, "in the non-governmental (teaching) institutions, the typical board member is associated with large-scale business, a banker, manufacturer, business executive, or prominent lawyer," to which, in the health sector, we could add a prominent physician. For instance, one study (41) showed that of the 734 trustees of 30 leading universities half were recognized members of the professions, and half were proprietors, managers, and bankers. Incidentally, let me add that it is quite misleading to assume that the class and corporate role of such board members is a passive one or that their function is that of rubber stamping what the administrators and medical faculty decide. In fact, their assumed passivity is one of delegated control. Actually, it was none other than Flexner (42) who, in a not very frequently quoted part of one of his reports, said that "the influence of the board of trustees . . . determines in the social and economic realms an atmosphere of timidity which is not without effect on critical appointments and promotions." Indeed, concerning the highest decisions, theirs is the first and final voice. And their first role, as

Galbraith (43) has indicated, is to ensure that "the aims of higher education, of course, are to be attuned to the needs of the industrial (corporate) system" which is usually also referred to as the "private enterprise system." In 1961, Dr. Pusey (44), then the President of Harvard, made this quite explicit when he said in a remarkable speech that "the end of all academic departments . . . is completely directed towards making the *private enterprise system* continue to work effectively and beneficially in a very difficult world." This clearly ideological statement, from a supposedly unideological academic leader of a presumably unideological establishment, is meritorious for its clarity, conciseness, and straight-forwardness. In fact, this commitment, which is far more typical than atypical of our academic institutions and foundations, cannot be disassociated from the nature of the predominant membership of the corporate and business leaders in the boards of trustees of academia and foundations.[8] The function and purpose of this dominant influence in the boards of trustees is to perpetuate the sets of values that will optimize their collective benefits as class and as corporate interests.

Allow me to clarify here that I do not believe that there is monopoly control in the value-generating system. However, I do think that the system of influence and control in that system is highly skewed in favor of the corporate and financial value system. And this dominant influence is felt not only in universities, foundations, and institutions of higher learning, but also in most of the value-generating systems, from the media to all other instruments of communication (46). As Miliband (29, p. 238) says, all these value-generating systems do contribute to the

> . . . fostering of a climate of conformity, not by the total suppression of dissent, but by the presentation of views which fall outside the consensus as curious heresies, or, even more effectively, by treating them as irrelevant eccentricities, which serious and reasonable people may dismiss as of no consequence. This is very functional [for the system].

Actually, another indication of this dominance of corporate values can be seen in the present debate in academia on national health insurance. In spite of the "hot" debate as to what type and nature of national health insurance "Americans may choose," and in spite of the critical nature of comments about our health sector made by considerable sectors of academia and even the mass media, not one of the proposals and not one

[8]For an updated analysis of the backgrounds, roles, and educational attitudes of university trustees, see reference 45.

report in the media questions the sanctity of the private sector, nor its pattern of control of our health institutions. And a whole series of alternatives that would question the present pattern, such as different types of national health services as opposed to just national health insurance, are not even raised, or are quickly dismissed as being "un-American." The sanctity of "private enterprise values," however has more to do with the pattern of control of the value-generating system by the financial and corporate interests than with the genetic-biological structure of the American population. As Marcuse (47) has indicated, the success of the system is to make unthinkable the possibility of its alternatives.

The Control of the Health Distribution Institutions

The voluntary community hospitals are the largest component of the health distribution institutions. Analyzing the boards of trustees of these hospitals, one sees less predominance of the representatives of financial and corporate capital, and more of the upper-middle class, and primarily of the professionals—especially physicians—and representatives of the business middle class. Even here, the other strata and classes, the working class and lower-middle class, which constitute the majority of the U.S. population, are not represented. Not one trade union leader (even a token one), for instance, sits on any board in the hospitals in the region of Baltimore (48). And, of course, even less represented on hospital boards are the unorganized workers. Figure 6 presents a summary of the percentage class distribution of the U.S. labor force, and how the classes are represented on the boards of the reproductive and distributive health institutions.

The False Dichotomy of Providers Versus Consumers

Out of the previous analysis it should be clear that I disagree with most of my colleagues who perceive the present basic dialectical conflict in the health sector of the United States—both in the financing and in the delivery of health services—to be between the consumers and the providers. To me this is a simplification that obfuscates the nature of the distribution of economic and political power in the United States today, both inside as well as outside the health sector. Although I would agree that the present delivery system seems to be controlled primarily by the providers and their different components, either the "patricians" or professionals of academia-based medicine, the practitioners or the

Figure 6
Estimated social class composition of the U.S. labor force
and of the boards of trustees of reproductive and delivery institutions
in the health sector

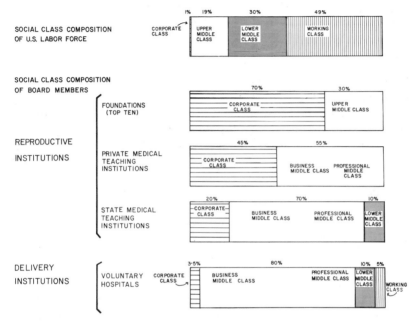

Sources: reference 45; V. Navarro, The control of the health institutions, Department of Health Care Organization, Johns Hopkins University, Baltimore (in process); and J. Pfeffer, Size, composition, and functions of hospital boards of directors: A study of organization-environment linkage. *Administrative Science Quarterly* 18(3): 349–364, 1973.

American Medical Association (AMA), and the hospital organizations or the American Hospital Association (AHA), I would disagree with the proposition that there is an inherent control given to them by their "unique" knowledge or that the situation cannot be changed. Actually, the power of the medical profession is delegated power. As Freidson (49) has indicated, "A profession attains and maintains its position by virtue of the protection and patronage of some elite segment of society which has been persuaded that there is some special value in its work." But as Frankenberg (50) has pointed out, this section or segment of the population is not so much an economic elite as a class, i.e. the corporate class described before. Remember, incidentally, that the Flexner Report and the first scientific medical schools were funded and subsidized by the enlightened establishment of the 1900s, i.e. the Rockefeller and Carnegie Foundations, the intellectual voices of the financial and corporate class of the early 1900s (51).

The great influence of the providers over the health institutions, which amounts to control of the health sector, is based on power delegated from other groups and classes, primarily the corporate class and the upper-middle class, to which the providers belong. Their specific interests may actually be in conflict with the power of other groups or strata within the upper-middle class and with the greater power of the corporate class. Indeed, as I have indicated elsewhere (52), the corporate powers of England and Sweden not only tolerated but even supported the nationalization of the health sector when the corporate interests required it, formalizing a dependency of the medical profession on those corporate and state interests.

To define the main dialectical conflict in the health sector as one of providers versus consumers assumes that (a) providers have the final and most powerful control of decision making in the health sector, and (b) consumers have a uniformity of interests, transcending class and other interests. Control of the health institutions, however, is primarily class control by the classes and groups described before, and only secondarily control by the professions. The dialectical conflicts that exist are not, then, between the providers and the consumers; but instead there is conflict (a) between the corporate class and the providers over the financing of the health sector, and (b) between the majority of the U.S. population, who belong to the working and lower-middle classes, and the controllers of the health delivery system—the corporate class and the upper-middle class, including the professionals.

The Corporate System and the State

Having described, however briefly, the patterns of influence in both the financing and the delivery systems of the health sector, let me address myself to the final question of our analysis, that of who has dominant influence over the state. Let me add right away that this is far from being a simple question.

Before I attempt to answer the question of who has dominant influence over the state, let me describe what I consider to be erroneous answers. One of these is that government is run by business. As a proponent of this theory put it, "Government and Congress are run by big business" (53). And actually, this idea is similar to Marx's statement in the *Communist Manifesto* (54) that "the state is the executive committee of the bourgeoisie." It is quite interesting, incidentally, that this view seems to have been held even by past presidents of the United States. Indeed, none other than President Woodrow Wilson said that "the masters of the government of the United States are the combined capitalists and manufacturers of the United States" (quoted in 32, p. 284). However, I find such statements too much of a simplification. But I find equally simplistic the idea, quite prevalent among our scholars, that the state organs are "above" business, or that business is even actually anti-government. I believe this explanation to be unhistorical and unempirical. Actually, in the executive branch of government:

> Businessmen were in fact the largest single occupational group in cabinets from 1889 to 1949; of the total number of cabinet members between these dates, more than 60 per cent were businessmen of one sort or another. Nor certainly was the business membership of American cabinets less marked in the Eisenhower years from 1953 to 1961. As for members of British cabinets between 1886 and 1950, close to one-third were businessmen, including three prime ministers—Bonar Law, Baldwin and Chamberlain. Nor again have businessmen been at all badly represented in the Conservative cabinets which held office between 1951 and 1964 (29, pp. 56–57).

In respect to the legislative branch, in 1970, as Hunt and Sherman (32, p. 288) point out:

> A total of 102 congressmen held stock or well-paying executive positions in banks or other financial institutions; 81 received regular income from law firms that generally represented big businesses. Sixty-three got their income from stock in the top defense contractors; 45, in the giant (federally regulated) oil and gas industries; 22, in radio and television companies; 11, in commercial airlines; and 9, in railroads. Ninety-eight congressmen were involved in numerous capital-gains transactions; each of them netted a profit of over $5,000 (and some as high as $35,000).

It is, therefore, difficult to conclude from these figures that businessmen are anti-government. Let me add that these businessmen in the corridors of power may not necessarily think of themselves as business representatives holding state power. But, it is highly unlikely, as Miliband says, that their vision of national interest runs against the interests of the business community. Indeed, values and beliefs do not change when the call of government takes place. The appointment of businessmen to positions of power has also been the practice in the federal health establishment. For instance, out of the last twelve Secretaries of Health, nine have had business backgrounds.

On the other hand, in the dichotomy between business and labor, labor leaders have been a small, very small minority indeed in the key positions of either the executive or legislative branch. Let me add, though, that this situation is far from unique to the United States. In Sweden, painted as a socialist heaven by some and as a hell by others, the number of workers' sons and daughters among the top Swedish politico-bureaucratic echelons was less than 9 per cent in 1961 (55).

This heavy involvement of businessmen in government, then, makes one begin to question the widely held belief that businessmen are against government. But, on the other hand, this involvement in, and heavy influence on, the state should not lead to the opposite conclusion that businessmen are the government—or at least not in the way that the land-owning aristocracy was the government in the 18th century. Indeed, sharing the power of government with big business are other groups who represent different interests. In the executive branch of the federal health establishment, for example, powerful groups with whom the businessmen share power are the professionals of academic medicine—the patricians— and, to a lesser degree, the practitioners. These two groups, while they are not the top decision makers (who are usually businessmen), do control the next-to-top echelons of policy in the executive of the federal health establishment, e.g. they are the Assistant Secretaries of Health and below. The medical practitioners, who control the AMA, incidentally, tend to be more influential on the legislative branch of the federal government than on the executive. An example, among many others, showing the differing degrees of influence the AMA has over the two branches of government, is the recent decision of Congress to follow the AMA's wishes and exclude the health sector from cost controls despite the very strong opposition to this exclusion from the executive branch. Still another example is that the AMA proposal for national health insurance is the one proposal with most sponsors in the Congress. And this selective attention by some members of the Congress is not without rewards. Actually, the Common Cause list of federal legislators who received AMA contributions during the last national election in 1972 (56) reads like a "Who's Who" of the health sector in the U.S. Congress.

There is indeed a diversity of interests in the health sector. Yet within this diversity that determines the plurality of sources of power in the federal establishment, there is a uniformity that unites these groups and sets them apart from other groups who do not share the basic characteristics, i.e. their social origin, education, and class situation. As Professor Matthews (57) notes:

> Those American political decision-makers for whom this information is available are, with very few exceptions, sons of professional men, proprietors and officials, and farmers. A very small minority are sons of wage-earners, low salaried workers, farm laborers or tenants . . . the narrow base from which political decision-makers appear to be recruited is clear.

In fact, the large majority of the governing classes belong, by social origin and by previous occupation, to our corporate and upper-middle classes, as defined before.

Let me underline, once again, that I am not implying that the corporate class and the upper-middle class, which predominate in and dominate the corridors of power, act and behave uniformly on the political scene. Indeed, they represent a plurality of interests that determines what is usually referred to as the political pluralism of our society. This plurality is reflected in the different programs put forward by the main political parties. In that respect, it is far from my intention to imply that all proposals for national health insurance, for example, are the same, or that they represent the same groups. Differences *do* exist. Yet the nature of this political pluralism means that the benefits of the system are consistently skewed in favor of those classes mentioned before. Moreover, the political debate which reflects that pluralism takes place within a common understanding and acceptance of certain basic premises and assumptions, which consistently benefit some classes more than others.

Let me add that this situation is not so much because of personalities, but because of the inner logic of the system, i.e. it is a syndrome of the distribution of economic and political power within our system. It is because of this inner logic that, when there is government intervention, the possible benefits of that intervention are not randomly distributed, but are largely very predictable. And the answer to the question of *cui bono?* to whom the goods? is predictably easy. Let me give you an example—that of the fiscal policies in general and of taxation in particular. Titmuss (58) in Britain and Kolko (59) in this country have shown that the two countries' systems of taxation have not weakened the income inequalities in either country but have actually accentuated them. A similar example in the health sector is the system of funding of most of the national health insurance proposals, which for the most part share the common denominator of being regressive (60).

With this introduction, let me describe, as I perceive them, the roles of state intervention as they relate to the health sector.[9] And I postulate that these roles are (a) the legitimization and defense of the private enterprise system, and (b) the strengthening of that system. These categories are somewhat artificial, and thus their separation is more one of convenience than of necessity.

The Legitimization and Defense of the System

According to Weber, the first role of any state is to assure the survival of the economic system. Thus, the main role of the state is the legitimization of the economic and political relationship via the different mechanisms at the state's disposal. These mechanisms range from the exclusive use of force, i.e. the armed forces and police, to the creation of social services, including the development of health services, with very many mechanisms of intervention between these alternatives. Actually, it was none other than Bismarck, the midwife of the welfare state, who first used the social insurance mechanism as a way of co-opting the forces threatening to the capitalist system of that time (61). Social security legislation was passed in England and other countries for similar reasons.

Nor are we strangers to this mechanism in this country. Piven and Cloward (62) have shown, for example, how welfare rolls are—and always have been—raised to reduce unrest among the poor. It was the function of welfare programs to integrate those sectors of the population who felt increasingly alienated from the political system and to give them the feeling of being a part of the system in which those programs were introduced. As Moynihan has indicated for the anti-poverty programs of the sixties, "They were intended to do no more than ensure that persons excluded from the political process in the South and elsewhere could nevertheless *participate* in the benefits of the community action programs. . . ." (quoted in 62, p. 268).

In that respect, the lateness of the United States to come to the welfare state stage may be due to the lack of pressure, primarily on the corporate class, from any force that could obtain a concession from that class and achieve what the European Left has achieved for its constituents. The potential for threat does exist, however, and the perception of that potential is explicitly manifested in a continuous call

---

[9]The roles of the state intervention, both inside and outside the health sector, are analyzed in greater detail in my paper "Social Class, Political Power and the State: Their Implications in Medicine," which is included in this volume.

for "law and order," and in expressed concern for the disintegration of the system. Indeed, the percentage of the American people who have expressed alienation from, and disillusionment with, their present system of government has achieved a record high in the history of the United States. A possible response by government to that popular alienation could be the establishment of measures such as income maintenance or national health insurance, aimed at integrating that alienated population into the political system. As the daily press has indicated, the increased attention of Presidents Nixon and Ford to the national health insurance issue on the political scene and the broadening of benefits, could easily be related to their concern with the alienation of the population from them personally and from the political system in general (63).

The Strengthening of the Private Enterprise System

In creating a welfare state, however, the inner logic of the system, which is a product of the pattern of economic and political power as explained before, determines that the distribution of benefits brought about through that state intervention is likely to benefit some groups more than others. Actually, it is because I believe the system functions in this way that I am skeptical—as are others—that national health insurance will solve what is usually referred to as the "health crisis" in this country. As Bodenheimer rightly points out, it is far from clear whose crisis national health insurance is supposed to solve—that of the financial interests of the insurance industry and of the providers themselves or that of the availability and accessibility needs of the majority of the population. Not surprisingly, after making a comprehensive analysis of the flow of funds in the health sector, Bodenheimer (60) postulates that:

> Just as federal defense appropriations subsidize the military-industrial complex, national health insurance will subsidize the medical-industrial complex.

Let me finish now by underlining, once again, that state intervention is not uniform, since it depends on the interests of the dominant group in the area in dispute. This is shown by the fact that each one of the different power groups in the health sector has put forward its own proposal aimed at optimizing its own interests. Thus, each proposal has a rationale and ideology behind it which respond to the specific economic interests of its proponents. And, again, reflecting the power of the insurance industry, all proposals, except one, have allowed and even encouraged the involvement of insurance in the health sector, with state subsidization of the private insurance industry. As Fein (64) has indicated in commenting on the Administration proposal, it is part and parcel of that proposal's strategy to strengthen the private market in health sector economic affairs. The passing of this proposal, as well as the majority of the others, would strengthen the contractual segment of the state sector that I discussed in a previous section. Indeed, as you may recall, following the categories outlined by O'Connor and Galbraith, I divided the state sector into two subsectors: the contractual part, in which the state contracts with and subsidizes the private sector, primarily the monopolistic or planned sector (such as in the case of the defense industry), and the part that is owned and operated by the public sector per se, with services that are owned and run by the state, such as the public health services.

The first subsector, or contractual one, would be strengthened with the passing of the suggested national health insurance, and would further expand what O'Connor calls the social-industrial complex. The rationale for that involvement, as *Fortune* magazine says, is that

> Implicit in the governmental appeals for help at all levels is an acknowledgement that large corporations are the major repository of some rather special capabilities that are now required. Business executives are increasingly identified as the most likely organizers of community-action programs, like the Urban Coalition and its local counterparts. Corporate managers often have the special close-quarters knowledge that enables them to visualize opportunities for getting at particular urban problems—e.g., the insurance companies' plans for investments in the slums. Finally, the new "systems engineering" capabilities of many corporations have opened up some large possibilities for dealing with just about any complex social problem (quoted in 27, pp. 55–56).

Medicare and Medicaid have already begun the expansion of the contractual subsector, and the rate of this expansion has established a record for the rate of growth of financial capital in this country. Indeed, from 1970 to 1973 the profits of the private health insurance industry increased by 120 per cent, establishing an all-time record (65,66).

Another objective of all the national health insurance proposals is to socialize the increasing costs of health insurance, and to stop the increased drain of funds that health costs represent for both capital and labor. In 1966, for example, contributions to health insurance plans exceeded $8 billion, and represented about 40 per cent of total fringe benefit costs (27, p. 142).

The other subsector of the state sector, the public sector (city hospitals, public health service hospitals, and others), will have the responsibility of taking care of the load that is considered unprofitable or less profitable by the private sector. As Roemer and Mera (67) have concisely shown, the patient population of our city hospitals consists for the most part of patients unwanted by the private sector. Thus, in the health sector, there occurs what happens in other sectors. It is the perceived function of the state to strengthen the private sector, through contracts and subsidies, and by taking care of the unwanted responsibilities of the private sector.

In summary, then, the defined patterns of dominance within the organs of the state explain and ensure that state intervention is aimed at (a) legitimizing those patterns of dominance, and (b) strengthening the private sector, and, of course, the groups that have dominance within it. And it is within this context of the functions and goals of state intervention that the debate regarding the different health insurance proposals must be understood. Thus, the arguments of the proponents of the various alternatives are designed to convince the average citizen that the proposed insurance will improve his or her life, and at the same time, to prove that the system is basically responsive to his or her needs. Yet, by the very nature of class dominance within the state, this intervention will predictably benefit some social classes, some economic groups, and some interest groups more than others.

Indeed, that the proposals are likely to benefit certain social classes more than others can be seen by the proposed system of funding in the majority of national health insurance proposals, based for the most part on either payroll taxes, social security taxes, and/or premiums, or a combination of these—all of them systems of funding that are highly regressive (60). Also, the likely benefit of these proposals to primarily the dominant economic groups in our society is clear in that the majority of proposals rely on the insurance industry to administer the national insurance scheme, thereby guaranteeing not only the continuation of but also a dramatic increase in the flow of money through that industry. The awareness of this possibility by the insurance industry undoubtedly explains the $9 million campaign that the health and life insurance industry budgeted for 1974 and 1975 to "educate" our citizenry, through TV and other media, on the "merits" of having the insurance industry "involved in and responsible for" the administration of the proposed national health insurance schemes (68).

Also, the provider interest groups will likely benefit to a large extent from whatever form of proposal may pass, sometimes sharing those benefits with the insurance industry, and sometimes competing with it for those benefits.

Thus, it is basically the patterns of dominance that condition the possibilities for change and the definitions of what is possible. Within these definitions and within these possibilities for change, it is unlikely, for example, that the funding of whatever insurance that may pass will be progressive, i.e. designed to ensure that the larger burden of the funding will fall on the strongest rather than the weakest shoulders. Also, within the defined boundaries of what is possible and what is not, it is highly improbable, whatever system of control and regulation may evolve, that the patterns of governance of our health institutions will change profoundly and become more responsive and accountable to the majority of those who either work in or are being served by those institutions. And, meanwhile, as all the "political drama and political heat" continue, the life of the average citizen is likely to remain the same. He is likely to repeat the old adage that "the more things change, the more they remain the same."

Conclusion

In summary, then, I have tried to show how the same economic and political forces that determine the class structure of the United States also determine the nature and functions of the U.S. health sector. Indeed, the composition, nature, and functions of the latter are the result of the degree of ownership, control, and influence that primarily the corporate and the upper middle classes have on the means of production, reproduction, and legitimization of U.S. society. This interpretation runs contrary to the most prevalent interpretation, which assumes that the "shape and form" of the health sector is a result of American values that prevail in all areas and spheres of American life. But such an explanation assumes that values are the cause, and not, as I postulate, a symptom of the distribution of economic and political power in the United States. In fact, that explanation avoids the question of which groups and classes have a dominant influence on the value-generating system and maintain, perpetuate, and legitimize it. According to my interpretation, they are the very same groups and classes that have a dominant influence over the systems of production, reproduction, and legitimization in other areas of the economy, including the organs of the state.

Let me underline, once again, that I do not believe these groups to be uniform, nor their dominant influence to be equivalent to control. Actually, I find this distinction between dominant influence and control a key one that has a number of implications, primarily in the area of strategies for stimulating change. Indeed, there is a plurality of interests among groups and among classes that explains and determines the political pluralism apparent today in the United States. Competition does exist. And a strategist for change has to be aware of and sensitive to the diversity of interests reflected in political debate (52). However, the competition that supports this pluralism is consistently and unavoidably unequal, skewed, and biased in favor of the dominant groups and classes. To quote the excellent description Miliband (29, pp. 164–165) has made of this situation:

> There is competition, and defeats for powerful capitalist interests as well as victories. After all, David did overcome Goliath. But the point of the story is that David was smaller than Goliath and that the odds were heavily against him.

The degree of skewedness in the distribution of economic and political power, both outside and within the health sector, is, as I have tried to show in this presentation, very dramatic indeed. And at a time when much time and energy are spent in academia in debating what would be the most perfect model for the health sector, it might have a salutary effect to underline that more important than the shape of the final product is the issue of who dominates the process. Thus, a primary intent of this presentation has been to show that the presently debated questions of what services to provide, and for whom, will actually be determined by whoever is dominant in the process of defining those questions and of formulating those answers.

Indeed, I have attempted in this paper to put the tree—our health sector—within the setting of the forest—the economic and political structure of our nation. I am aware that I may have left very many areas loosely sketched or not defined at all, but I suppose there are risks in daring to face the totality. And needless to say, I am aware that this analysis is, according to present Parsonian standards of orthodoxy, an "unorthodox" one. But it may in the long term serve as one more effort to question that orthodoxy. Meanwhile, in the short run, I hope it will at least stimulate students of health services to look wider and deeper than just at their own health sector.

References

1. Mills, C.W. *The Sociological Imagination.* Grove Press, New York, 1959.

2. Birnbaum, N. *Toward a Critical Sociology.* Oxford University Press, New York, 1971.

3. Dreitzel, H.P. *On the Social Basis of Politics.* Macmillan Company, New York, 1969.

4. Coulson, M.A., and Riddell, C. *Approaching Sociology: A Critical Introduction.* Routledge and Kegan Paul, London, 1973.

5. Baran, P., and Sweezy, P. *Monopoly Capital,* pp. 2–3. Monthly Review Press, New York, 1968.

6. Kumpa, P.J. Hail to the middle class! *Baltimore Sun* pp. K1 and K3, March 10, 1974.

7. Bell, D. *End of Ideology: On the Exhaustion of Political Ideas in the Fifties.* Free Press, New York, 1960.

8. Parker, R. *The Myth of the Middle Class: Notes on Affluence and Equality.* Liveright, New York, 1972.

9. Horowitz, I.L., editor. *Power, Politics and People: The Collected Essays of C. Wright Mills,* p. 317. Oxford University Press, New York, 1962. (Quoted in R. Miliband, *The State in Capitalist Society: An Analysis of the Western System of Power,* p. 20. Weidenfeld and Nicolson, London, 1969.)

10. Irish, M., and Prothro, J. *The Politics of American Democracy,* p. 38. Prentice-Hall, Englewood Cliffs, N.J., 1965. (Quoted in E.K. Hunt and H.J. Sherman, *Economics: An Introduction to Traditional and Radical Views,* p. 284. Harper and Row, New York, 1972.)

11. Samuelson, P. *Economics,* Ed. 8, p. 110. McGraw-Hill Book Company, New York, 1972.

12. United States Congress. *Economic Report of the President, 1974.* U.S. Government Printing Office, Washington, D.C., 1974.

13. Shanahan, E. Income distribution found unchanged. *New York Times* p. 10, February 2, 1974.

14. Clark, J.B. *The Distribution of Wealth.* Macmillan Company, New York, 1924. (Quoted in B. Silverman and M. Yanowitch, Radical and liberal perspectives on the working class. *Social Policy* 4(4): 40–50, 1974.)

15. Rawls, J.A. *Theory of Justice.* Harvard University Press, Cambridge, Mass., 1971.

16. Barry, B. *The Liberal Theory of Justice: A Critical Examination of the Principal Doctrines in "A Theory of Justice" by John Rawls.* Clarendon Press, Oxford, 1972.

17. Silverman, B., and Yanowitch, M. Radical and liberal perspectives on the working class. *Social Policy* 4(4): 40–50, 1974.

18. Westergaard, J.H. Sociology: The myth of classlessness. In *Ideology in Social Science,* edited by R. Blackburn, pp. 119–163. Fontana, New York, 1972.

19. Bowles, S., and Gintis, H. IQ in the U.S. class structure. *Social Policy* 3(4 and 5): 65–96, 1973.

20. Simpson, M.A. *Medical Education: A Critical Approach.* Butterworths, London, 1972.

21. Robson, J. The NHS Company, Inc.? The social consequence of the professional dominance in the National Health Service. *Int. J. Health Serv.* 3(3): 413–426, 1973.

22. Kleinbach, G. Social structure and the education of health personnel. *Int. J. Health Serv.* 4(2): 297–317, 1974.

23. *Evidence of the Royal College of Surgeons to the Royal Commission on Doctors and Dentists Remuneration.* Her Majesty's Stationery Office, London, 1958. (Quoted in J. Robson, The NHS Company, Inc.? The social consequence of the professional dominance in the National Health Service. *Int. J. Health Serv.* 3(3): 413–426, 1973.)

24. Lyden, F.J., Geiger, H.J., and Peterson, O. *The Training of Good Physicians.* Harvard University Press, Cambridge, Mass., 1968. (Cited in M.A. Simpson, *Medical Education: A Critical Approach,* p. 35. Butterworths, London, 1972.)

25. Kleinbach, G. Social Class and Medical Education. Department of Education, Harvard University, Cambridge, Mass., 1974.

26. Mills, C.W. *The Power Elite,* p. 39. Oxford University Press, New York, 1956.

27. O'Connor, J. *The Fiscal Crisis of the State.* St. Martin's Press, New York, 1973.

28. Galbraith, J.K. *Economics and the Public Purpose.* Houghton-Mifflin Company, Boston, 1973.

29. Miliband, R. *The State in Capitalist Society: An Analysis of the Western System of Power.* Weidenfeld and Nicolson, London, 1969.

30. Bonnell, V., and Reich, M. *Workers and the American Economy: Data on the Labor Force.* New England Free Press, Boston, 1973.

31. Williams, G.A. Gramsci's concept of hegemonia. *Journal of the History of Ideas* 21(4):587, 1960.

32. Hunt, E.K., and Sherman, H.J. *Economics: An Introduction to Traditional and Radical Views.* Harper and Row, New York, 1972.

33. Committee on Government Operations of the United States Senate. *Disclosure of Corporate Ownership.* U.S. Government Printing Office, Washington, D.C., 1973.

34. Pattman Committee Staff Report for the Domestic Finance Subcommittee of the House Committee on Banking and Currency. *Commercial Banks and Their Trust Activities; Emerging Influence on the American Economy.* U.S. Government Printing Office, Washington, D.C., 1968.

35. Mintz, M. Eight institutions control most of top firms. *Washington Post* pp. A1 and A16, January 6, 1974.

36. Iglehart, J.K. National insurance plan tops ways and means agenda. *National Journal* 6(11): 387, 1974.

37. Bodenheimer, T., Cummings, S., and Harding, E. Capitalizing on illness: The health insurance industry. *Int. J. Health Serv.* 4(4): 569–584, 1974.

38. Health plan progress. Editorial. *New York Times* p. E16, April 7, 1974.

39. Kelman, S. Toward the political economy of medical care. *Inquiry* 8(3): 30–38, 1971.

40. MacIver, R.M. *Academic Freedom in Our Time,* p. 78. Gordian Press, New York, 1967. (Cited in R. Miliband, *The State in Capitalist Society: An Analysis of the Western System of Power,* p. 251. Weidenfeld and Nicolson, London, 1969.)

41. Beck, H.P. *Men Who Control Our Universities,* p. 51. King's Crown Press, London, 1947.

42. Flexner, A. *Universities: American, English, German,* p. 180. Oxford University Press, New York, 1930.

43. Galbraith, J.K. *The New Industrial State,* p. 370. Houghton-Mifflin Company, Boston, 1967.

44. Pusey, N.M. *Age of the Scholar: Observations on Education in a Troubled Decade,* p. 171. Harvard University Press, Cambridge, Mass., 1963.

45. Hartnett, R.T. College and university trustees: Their backgrounds, roles and educational attitudes. In *Crisis in American Institutions,* J. Skolnick and E. Currie, pp. 359–372. Little, Brown and Company, Boston, 1973.

46. Servan-Schreiber, J.L. *The Power to Inform: Media—The Business of Information.* McGraw-Hill Book Company, New York, 1974.

47. Marcuse, H. *Repressive Tolerance.* Beacon Press, Boston, 1972.

48. Van Gelder, P., leader of the Baltimore American Federation of Labor-Congress of Industrial Organizations (AFL-CIO). Personal communication.

49. Freidson, E. *Profession of Medicine: A Study of the Sociology of Applied Knowledge,* p. 72. Dodd, Mead, and Company, New York, 1970.

50. Frankenberg, R. Functionalism and after? Theory and developments in social science applied to the health field. *Int. J. Health Serv.* 4 (3): 411–427, 1974.

51. Berliner, H. A Larger Perspective on the Flexner Report. Johns Hopkins University, Baltimore. (In process.)

52. Navarro, V. A critique of the present and proposed strategies for redistributing resources in the health sector and a discussion of alternatives. *Med. Care* 12(9): 721–742, 1974.

53. Green, M.J., Fallows, J.M., and Zwick, D.R. *Who Runs Congress?* Ralph Nader Congress Project. Bantam Books, New York, 1972.

54. Marx, K., and Engels, F. *The Communist Manifesto.* International Publishing Company, New York, 1960.

55. Therborn, G. Power in the kingdom of Sweden. *International Socialist Journal* 2: 59, 1965.

56. *1972 Federal Campaign Finances. Business, Agriculture, Dairy and Health,* Vol. 1. Common Cause, Washington, D.C., 1974.

57. Matthews, D.R. *The Social Background of Political Decision Makers,* pp. 23–24. Doubleday, New York, 1954. (Quoted in R. Miliband, *The State in Capitalist Society: An Analysis of the Western System of Power,* p. 61. Weidenfeld and Nicolson, London, 1969.)

58. Titmuss, R. *Income Distribution and Social Change.* Allen and Unwin, Ltd., London, 1963.

59. Kolko, G. *Wealth and Power in America.* Praeger, New York, 1968.

60. Bodenheimer, T. Health care in the United States: Who pays? *Int. J. Health Serv.* 3(3): 427–434, 1973.

61. Rimlinger, G.V. *Welfare Policy and Industrialization in Europe, America and Russia.* John Wiley and Sons, New York, 1971.

62. Piven, F.F., and Cloward, R.A. *Regulating the Poor: The Functions of Public Welfare.* Vintage Books, New York, 1971.

63. Woodson, D.W. National health insurance: A big role reversal takes place in Congress. *Medical World News* 15(14): 69, 1974.

64. Fein, R. The new national health spending policy. *New Engl. J. Med.* 290(3): 137–140, 1974.

65. Glasser, M., Director of the Social Security Department of the United Automobile Workers of America (UAW). Personal communication.

66. Glasser, M. The Pros and Cons of the Private Insurance Involvement in the Health Sector. Paper presented at the Policy and Planning Seminar, School of Hygiene and Public Health, Johns Hopkins University, Baltimore, April 18, 1974.

67. Roemer, M.I., and Mera, J.A. "Patient-dumping" and other voluntary agency contributions to public agency problems. *Med. Care* 11(1): 30–39, 1973.

68. *Washington Report on Medicine and Health* No. 1407, p. 1, June 17, 1974.

The Labor Force: Women as Producers of Services in the Health Sector of the United States

Although women constitute a majority in our U.S. population, it was not until the early 1970s that the discriminatory conditions facing women became widely discussed and debated. And this discussion has emerged in all economic and social sectors, including the health one. Many articles have appeared translating this discussion. Still, most of the lengthy bibliography on the subject (documenting and analyzing the extent of sexism in the health sector) seems to focus on the problems faced by professional women. But, however important those problems may be, they are only a part—a small part at that—of the far greater problems encountered by all women who are producers of services in the health sector. The objectives of this article, then, are to (a) describe the situation of not only a few, but of all women who are producers of services in the health labor force, within the context of the overall labor force in the United States; (b) give my own interpretation of some of the factors that cause that situation; and (c) present a possible strategy for change.

In trying to understand the situation of women as producers of services in the health sector, we have to focus our analysis (a) not on the world of women, but on the world of men, and (b) not just on the health sector, but primarily on the socioeconomic forces of the overall society that determine the function, nature, and composition of that sector to begin with. Indeed, I believe that the failure of most sociological research to follow such an approach, and to focus instead just on women or just on the health sector, has led those studies to conclusions that have been empirically invalid and ineffective policy-wise. And because of their importance, let me discuss these two major weaknesses in greater detail.

The weakness of the first approach, i.e. focusing only on the situation of women, is that it fails to recognize that the so-called "women's question" or "women's problem" is actually the problem of men and society, i.e. to understand the present situation of women as producers in the health sector, we must also understand the distribution of political and economic power in the world of men. In this regard, current research on conditions faced by women is very similar to the numerous studies and analyses of poverty and the poor that were carried out in the 1960s, when poverty was "discovered" in the U.S. At that time, many studies were conducted on the poor themselves. Very few of these studies, however, examined the economic and political system which determined that poverty. And as a result of this singular focus, the strategies for improving the conditions of the poor were framed in terms of the poor themselves. Today, we have as many poor people—if not more—as when those strategies started.

In the 1970s, one can see a replication of this singular focus in the study of the so-called women's question, in which there is very little consideration of the social and economic systems, controlled by men of defined class backgrounds, which are responsible for the inferior social and economic status of working women. And just as poverty cannot be understood without an understanding of wealth, the distribution of wealth, and the reasons for the wealth and income differentials in this country, the situation of women in the health sector cannot be understood without an understanding of the world of men and the distribution of the social, economic, and political power within that world. To understand the situation of women, then, one must analyze not women as such (as if they themselves were responsible for their situation), but the entire socio-economic and political system that generates, creates, and perpetuates the present situation of women.

The second limitation of a large number of sociological studies of women as producers in the health sector has been their focus on the health sector itself, i.e. an analysis of the social forces within the health sector as determinants of the distribution of responsibilities within that sector. In doing so, however, an assumption is made that the health sector is autonomous and has a dynamic of its own. An example of this erroneous focus is the great "sales job" that is currently being done by a number of international agencies—including the World Health Organization—that are trying to apply the experience of the Chinese barefoot doctors in other developing and even developed countries. In this promotional activity, an interesting and positive element of the Chinese health services is assumed to be exportable to other countries as well. And yet, as the fascinating and candid account of a group of Iranian health workers who unsuccessfully tried to import and implant that Chinese experience to Iran indicates, that experience is not transferable to countries possessing different economic and political systems (1, p. 1331). Indeed, those exporters seem to be unaware that the very creative and imaginative use of personnel implied in the barefoot doctors' experiences in the People's Republic of China assumes and subsumes a series of political, economic and social values that are more the exception than the rule in the countries that are trying to duplicate those experiences.

The increased attempts to replicate in this country the successful

Chinese and Cuban movements of self-reliance and self-care reflect a similar lack of awareness that those movements in those countries do not have an autonomy of their own, but rather are part and parcel of broader political and social forces that determine and explain the composition, nature and functions of those movements—broader political and social forces, I may add, that are for the most part absent in our society.

Let me clarify here that none of my comments should be understood as a note of skepticism about the learning value of international studies, or international conferences for that matter. Rather, they are made with the intention of stimulating a broadening of those studies and conferences to include the analysis of the tree—the present situation of women as producers in the health sector—within the comprehension of the forest— the distribution of social, economic and political power in those societies.

Sex, Class and Occupational Structure of the U.S. Labor Force

Let us begin, then, with an analysis of the distribution of social, economic and political power in our society, starting with an analysis of the class, sex and occupational structure of our population and our labor force. As I have indicated in previous articles, the most important sectors of economic life in our society are controlled by a very small number of people (less than 2 per cent of the population), who constitute the upper or corporate class. These are the owners and/or managers of a markedly disproportionate share of the personal wealth and their income (averaging $80,000–100,000 yearly) is largely derived from this ownership. Only 0.1 per cent of the corporate owners and managers are female. At the other end of the social class structure, there is the working class, composed primarily of industrial or blue-collar workers (20 per cent of which are women), workers in the services sector (83 per cent women), and agricultural wage earners (3.3 per cent female).

Between these two extremes, there is the middle class which consists of (a) professionals, of which 10 per cent are women; (b) businessmen (1.3 per cent female); (c) self-employed shopkeepers and craftsmen (28 per cent female); and (d) clerical and sales workers, of which 82.6 per cent are women. Groupings (a) and (b) of this category are generally classified as the upper-middle class, and groups (c) and (d) as the lower-middle class. It is worth noting that the lower-middle class is closely related to the working class in terms of income, status and life style. This is strengthened by the fact that about one-half of all female clerical and sales workers are married to working class men.

Sex, Class and Occupational Structure of the U.S. Health Labor Force

This class, sex and occupational structure is also reflected in the composition of those who participate in the health sector. At the top of that sector, we find the physicians, whose annual median income of $40,000 places them in the top 5 per cent of our society. Mainly of upper-middle class backgrounds, physicians are overwhelmingly male (92.1 per cent) and white. Incidentally, only one other country in the Western developed world—Spain—has a lower percentage of women among the professional health labor force. Far below this upper class layer in the health sector are the paraprofessionals, equivalent in terms of income to the lower-middle class clerical/sales workers grouping in the overall labor force. Comprised of nurses, physical and occupational therapists, technicians, etc., this group is primarily female (i.e. 97.3 per cent of registered nurses, 69.6 per cent of technicians, and 76 per cent of therapists are women). Below this group is the majority of the labor force in the health sector—the auxiliary, ancillary and service personnel—whose annual median income was $4,000 in 1970. This grouping is predominantly female (84.1 per cent), includes a disproportionate number of blacks (30 per cent), and represents the working class within the health sector.

It is interesting to note that the income differentials among these groups have increased very dramatically over time. From 1949 to 1970, the growth in the approximate annual net median income was from $17,000 to $44,000 for general surgeons, $12,000 to $42,000 for internists, $12,000 to $37,000 for general practitioners (2), and $6,000 to $27,000 for dentists (3 and 4). During the same period, however, the approximate annual gross median income grew from $2,400 to $5,800 for paramedicals, and from $1,300 to $3,500 for service workers (5 and 6).

This analysis demonstrates that within the labor force in the health sector, women constitute the majority of all producers—a majority concentrated in the lower-middle class and working class echelons of the labor force. It is for this reason that sex and class are clearly intertwined for most, though not all, women in the health sector. The analysis of the whys of the situations of women in the health sector is thus closely related to the analysis of the class composition of the health sector.

The Economic Structure of the U.S.

To explain these variations in the sex, class and occupational structure of
the labor force, within as well as outside the health sector, we first have to
look at the three main sectors of the economy, i.e. monopolistic, competitive and state, described in the preceding article.[1] There, we saw that
the health labor force has the characteristics of the competitive sector,
which is composed of the business middle class, small percentages of blue
and white-collar workers, and a large percentage of service workers,
primarily auxiliary and ancillary personnel. This sector—a declining one
in contemporary society—is labor-intensive (as opposed to capital-
intensive), poorly paid, predominantly female and poorly unionized.

Both the health services and the competitive sector are supportive to
the main sector of the U.S. economic structure—the monopolistic sector.
The latter sector (which includes large financial and corporate capital) is
the one which has the dominant influence over the economic and political
institutions in our country, and this influence extends to the health institutions as well. Moreover, the nature and composition of the supportive services are largely determined by the needs of that sector. The
consequences of this relationship, in which the health services are both
supportive and dependent, are many. But a major one is the feminization
of the labor force of the supportive sectors (such as the competitive
sector) and of the supportive services (including health services).

The Whys of Sex Discrimination in the Health Sector

Among the factors that explain the situation of women, I would single out
the social and economic role of the family in our society as a main
determinant of the skewed division of labor in the economy in general,
and in the health sector in particular. Indeed, according to the distribution of responsibilities within the family, the main function of the
husband is to be an active member of the labor force and the agent of
production. The wife, on the other hand, is responsible for maintaining
(caring for) and reproducing the family. A result of this distribution of
responsibility (and one rarely acknowledged) is that although the
employer pays for the work of one person, he actually gets the work of
two. If employers paid for the housewife's work (facilitating the husband's

[1]The sectors of the U.S. economy are described in detail in "An Explanation of the
Composition, Nature and Functions of the Present Health Sector in the United States" (pp.
135–169 in this volume), as is the sex, class and occupational structure of the health
labor force.

participation in the labor force), considerable economic cost would be incurred—cost that is now completely avoided. Instead, the only compensation for this work is what are usually referred to as the "emotional rewards" that the wife is supposed to derive from working and caring for her family. This "emotional rewards philosophy," along with the division of labor within the family, primarily benefits the employers in society who, again, pay for the work of one and get the work of two.

Another socioeconomic factor that in part explains the division of labor within the family is the usefulness for the economic system of having a reserve army of workers, i.e. women who work at home for the most part but whose value to the economy as workers outside the home depends on the need for labor within the economy. Thus, during periods of labor shortages, women are encouraged to move into the labor force, but when there is widespread unemployment (as there is now), the political and economic structure hinders rather than encourages entry and involvement of women in the labor force. No doubt, the lack of receptivity of both the Nixon and Ford Administrations towards the creation of day-care centers in this country can be explained, to a large degree, by the fear of further exacerbating the unemployment situation.

These two socio-economic factors, among others, explain the social and economic usefulness of the present division of labor within the family, with the "woman's work" being primarily at home. Moreover, this very division of labor and the values that support it are continually reinforced and perpetuated by all the systems of communication and education in this country. Both are aimed at sustaining what Galbraith terms the convenient social virtues (7, p. 30), i.e. virtues that are supported by the powerful in society. And one of these is the merit ascribed to the woman who is a good homemaker. To be otherwise is to have it said she is "neglecting her home and family, i.e. her real work. She ceases to be a woman of acknowledged virtue" (7, p. 32).

The division of roles found in the family also appears in the health sector, with the predominantly upper class, white, male physicians being, according to the conventional wisdom, the unquestioned leaders of the health team; the nurses and paraprofessionals, predominantly female, the dependents and appendages to the physicians; and the auxiliary and ancillary personnel, predominantly female and working class by definition, at the bottom and supportive to all. Actually, this set of relations was perceived in just this light by none other than Florence Nightingale, who saw the characteristics of the nurse as those of providing wifely support to the physician, motherly devotion to the patient, and firm but kind discipline to the attendants and auxiliaries (8, pp. 34–35). And an example of ways the media reinforces these role definitions and the values that support them is the most popular television program in the United States dealing with health care— "Marcus Welby," in which all the MDs on the show are male, upper class, and thoughtful and compassionate, with the nurses presented as nice, sweet females who are appendages to the physician.

Given these social and economic needs of the system, it is quite logical that women are the majority of workers in a sector whose main function within the economy is to provide care to and maintenance of the population, and it is also logical that, within that sector, women tend to perform the conditional and dependent jobs. This situation, briefly described above, is found not only in the social and economic spheres of society, but also in the political ones. This can be illustrated by reviewing the sex and class composition of the decision-making bodies (boards of trustees) of institutions in the health sector, where, as indicated in Figure 1, there is very low representation of both women and the lower-middle and working classes—the majority of the United States population. The majority of producers, both in the health sector and in the rest of society, are practically nonexistent in the corridors of power. And in the health sector, most of those producers are women. A similar situation appears in the different agencies of government involved in the health sector, where corporate leaders and representatives of the professional and business upper-middle class, most of them males, predominate.

A Possible Strategy for Change

From this analysis of the sex and class structure of the labor force, both outside and within the health sector, it should be clear that it is highly unlikely that any profound and meaningful changes will take place for the benefit of the majority and not just a minority of women—and men—in the health sector unless the patterns of control of that sector change, with a change in the sex and class composition and the system of governance of the agencies in the health sector and its institutions.

It should be emphasized, however, that the inclusion of women in the corridors of power of our institutions is a necessary but not a sufficient condition for improving the situation of the majority of women in the health sector. Thus, I believe that the appearance of women in positions of power in the health sector will serve to improve the positions of women

Figure 1

Estimated Social Class and Sex Composition of U.S. Labor
Force, Health Labor Force, and Boards of Trustees of Reproductive and
Delivery Institutions in the Health Sector

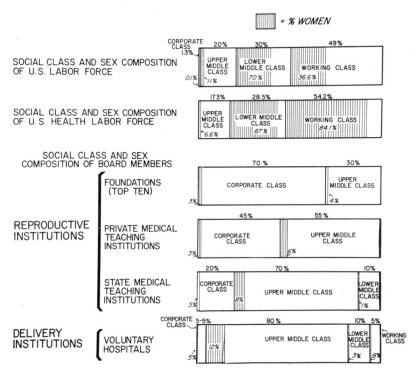

in that sector in general only to the extent that these women are representative of and accountable to the workers in the sector as a whole, the
majority of whom are lower-middle and working class women. I
emphasize this point because it has been my experience that when the
boards of trustees of health institutions, controlled so far by the city
fathers, expand to include the city mothers, the situations of the majority
of our citizens, the city orphans, do not improve. Indeed, the betterment
of a few does not imply, nor does it result in, the betterment of the many.
Another example of this is that while the number of women among
medical students has increased very substantially in recent years, the
percentage of women—and men—in these schools from working class

and lower-middle class families has remained constant over the last sixty years (9)! Class discrimination is indeed the most persistent, continuous and least discussed of all forms of discrimination.

Moreover, experience indicates that class loyalties are far stronger than sex loyalties. For example, in terms of socioeconomic behavior, the female physician is far closer to and supportive of the male physician than she is to the cleaning women in the hospital. Similarly, other oppressed groups in this country, such as blacks, are finding out that the broadening of opportunity for the black upper-middle class has not resulted in the betterment of the situation of the majority of the blacks in this country, whose oppression continues undiminished. Indeed, to limit the concern of women's liberation, black liberation or any other liberation movement to the fight for the advancement of those belonging to the upper and upper-middle classes leads merely to a change in the sex or racial composition of those at the top, leaving conditions for those at the bottom unchanged.

In summary, if our concern is for the fate and life of the majority of women in our society, then our strategy should be one of making women's liberation part and parcel of an authentic *human* liberation, where our society will be designed to benefit the many, and not just the few. And the betterment of the many will be related to the degree that the many are represented in the sources and corridors of power, presently controlled by the few. It is because of this that the demand for the rights of women in the health sector is intrinsically related to the demand for a more democratic, representative, and accountable system than we have today. It is this broader struggle that will finally give the majority of women, and men, in our population—those in the working and lower-middle classes—control over the institutions they support, work for, and pay for. As Mother Jones, that great trade union leader among the Appalachian miners said, "It is to break with the control that the few have over our lives, that we need the work and the struggle of all of us." And it is in terms of this understanding that the struggle for women's liberation also implies the struggle for the liberation of us all.

References

1. Ronaghy, H.A. Solter, S. Is the Chinese "barefoot doctor" exportable to rural Iran? *Lancet* 1 (7870), 1974.

2. The Survey of Physicians. *Medical Economics.* Oradell, New Jersey, 1972.

3. Dentists' incomes surveyed by Commerce Department. *Journal of the American Dental Association* 45: 248, 1952.

4. 1971 survey of dental practice III. Income of dentists by type of practice, personnel employed, and other factors. *Journal of the American Dental Association* 84: 636–639, 1972.

5. United States Bureau of the Census. *Census of Population: 1970. Subject Reports: Final Report PC (2)–7A, Occupational Characteristics.* Government Printing Office, Washington, D.C., 1973.

6. United States Bureau of the Census. *Census of Population: 1950. Vol. 2, Characteristics of the Population, Part 1, Summary, Chapter C.* Government Printing Office, Washington, D.C., 1953.

7. Galbraith, J.K. *Economics and the Public Purpose.* Houghton Mifflin, Boston, 1973.

8. Ehrenreich, B. and English, D. *Witches, Midwives, and Nurses: A History of Women Healers.* The Feminist Press, Old Westbury, N. Y., 1973.

9. Kleinbach, G. *Social Class and Medical Education.* Department of Education, Harvard University (in preparation).

PART IV:
CLASS, POLITICAL POWER,
AND HEALTH CARE

Social Class, Political Power, and the State: Their Implications in Medicine

> To those with whom I share a praxis aimed at converting the state "from an organ superimposed upon society into one completely subordinated to it." (Karl Marx, *Critique of the Gotha Program*)

INTRODUCTION

According to the means of communication in contemporary capitalist societies, our Western system of power is in a state of crisis. Editorial after editorial appears in the prominent press under variations of the title "What Has Gone Wrong?" And in the quest for answers to this disquieting question, there has emerged an increasing awareness that most of the accepted explanations in the Western system of thought on the nature of our societies are either erroneous or seriously insufficient. Consequently, a rekindling of old theories, as well as a presentation of new ones, is appearing in the realm of a debate that aims at providing alternative explanations of our realities. And in this search for alternatives, concerns about the distribution of political power, the legitimacy of our political systems, and the nature of the state are very much in the center of debate. This work is an attempt to contribute to that debate.

Divided into three sections, Section I presents a critique of contemporary theories of the Western system of power. The first half discusses the well established countervailing pluralist and power elite theories, as well as those of bureaucratic and professional control, and is followed in the second half with a critique of those Marxist theories that have most frequently been debated in present times, i.e. economic determinism, structural determinism, and corporate statism.

In the majority of this last group of theories, the state is considered to be much in the center of understanding our reality. Thus, the role, nature, characteristics, and mode of the state intervention is the subject of Section II. In this section, I aim at developing a Marxist theory of the state, building upon current debate, which has been greatly enriched by the contributions of Gramsci and of Miliband, Offe, Gough, O'Connor, Poulantzas, Althusser, and others, to all of whom I am in great intellectual debt.

A component of the analysis of political power and of the nature of the state that is greatly underdeveloped is the study of the modus operandi of the state, the subject of Section III. In this section, I present an expansion of that analysis, with specific focus on the mode of state intervention in contemporary developed capitalist societies, taking medicine as the arena of exposition. Also, I try, in this section, to explain the why of the dramatic growth of state intervention in the health sector, with an added analysis of the dialectical relationship between that growth and the current fiscal crisis of the state. Both are intrinsically and dialectically related.

In all three sections, I have focused on Western European countries and on North America, choosing many of my examples and categories from the area of medicine. The reason for the former is primarily biographical. In the course of my experience, I have lived in several Western European countries, as well as in the U.S., and it is from these societies that most of my political practice derives and where most of my theory focuses. As for my choice, in many instances, of medicine as an area for studying the nature of our society, of political power, and of the state, this flows from my belief that medicine is a much mystified area, subject, and sector in our societies and one where Marxist analyses and scrutinies have been few and far between.

SECTION I:

A CRITIQUE OF CONTEMPORARY THEORIES OF
THE WESTERN SYSTEM OF POWER

The Assumed Homogenization of Contemporary Western Societies

The most prevalent explanation that appears in economic, political and sociological analyses of the nature of contemporary Western societies is that, as a result of welfare state policies, social mobility and an enlargement of opportunities, these societies are being recast in a mold of middle class conditions and life styles that obviates their characterization as class societies and falsifies their designation as capitalist ones. Indeed, it is simply assumed and presented as a statement of fact that, because of welfare state and Keynesian economic policies, a substantial redistribution of wealth and income has taken place in those societies, with a progressive narrowing in the inequalities of consumption and an increasing broadening of opportunities for individual advancement. To that effect, an extensive literature has appeared to demonstrate the narrowing and even disappearance of class differentials in the consumption of goods and services, including health services, in our societies. For example, in a popular and influential volume on the British National Health Service (NHS), Cochrane (1) indicates that because of the NHS, differences in the consumption of medical care by social class have virtually disappeared in Great Britain. He takes Titmuss (2) and Tudor Hart (3) to task for their undue concern with class inequalities because, according to him, there are far more important inequities to worry about (4). Similarly, Bice and others (5) have postulated that in the U.S., Medicaid and other anti-poverty programs have rendered class differentials in medical care consumption a thing of the past. And if any differences do exist, they are more likely to be skewed in favor of the lower than the upper echelons of our social spectrum. Actually, in what is held to be the most thorough and best known analysis of equity in the health sectors in the U.K., the U.S., and Sweden, social class as a cause of cleavage and of differential consumption is neither considered nor even mentioned (6).

Such analyses assume that, contributing to this homogenization of consumption, there is a process of social fluidity and mobility so open and all-encompassing that distinctions between classes are being blurred as never before, making the whole category of class irrelevant. In the process, social heredity and birth are dramatically weakened as explanatory variables of success, while merit and learning—and perhaps just a little bit of luck—become the passwords for access to the ever increasing number of new opportunities. As one of the main theorists of this paradigm indicates, Western developed societies are

> relatively open so that an individual or group is able to find its niche in society in some reasonable relationship to its efforts, ability, and aspirations within the accepted rules of the game (7).

Because of this homogenization and the opportunities it has engendered, the working class and what used to be its chronic underconsumption of goods and services has, for all practical purposes, vanished to become part of a much larger middle class which embraces the bulk of our Western populations. For some, like Anderson, that process started decades ago when the middle class was (and still is)

> the source of entrepreneurial, technical, and managerial skills, which exploited natural resources, developed the economy, and thus began to create a social surplus that spilled over into other endeavors such as the arts, education, health services, and warring for national honor and expansion (8).

The transformation of society into a middle class society does not imply, of course, that there has been a complete homogenization of consumption. But while these writers recognize that some sectors of society, i.e. the poor, remain marginal, it is assumed that for them as well, this marginality is both provisional and correctable.[1]

It is further assumed that the process of homogenization has been accompanied and even facilitated by a change in the values in our societies that has reflected the disappearance of class consciousness. Values and ethos such as individual achievement, hard drive, competitiveness and family security—values usually identified with the middle class—are held to have also become widely accepted by manual workers. Thus, class consciousness is increasingly being replaced by a concern for status and for a middle class pattern of consumption. And, as Westergaard has indicated, "In this psychological analysis of class perceptions . . . loyalties of the world of work are replaced by loyalties of the hearth" (9). Furthermore, this vanishing of class consciousness is supposed to be accompanied by a dilution and disappearance of the working class culture. The working class itself has thus practically disappeared, having been absorbed by and become part and parcel of our middle class or mass society.

It is worth noting that the above interpretation of our societies' reality is prevalent not only in conservative and liberal circles,[2] but also among large sectors of the Left. For example, most of the analysts of the Frankfurt School in Europe (10), and Marcuse (11) and Aronowitz (12) in the U.S., have expressed the belief that the working class in developed capitalist societies, which they once saw as the only potential leverage for change, has lost that potential and instead been absorbed into society as merely a part of the larger consuming masses. Those masses, they say, are concerned mainly with a narrow personal interest in consumption, have become politically apathetic, and are being manipulated by the ruling or corporate elite. And according to these writers on the Left, the distribution, nature, and composition of our resources—including medical resources—are not so much a result of class struggle—a passé category of concern only to "vulgar" Marxists—but more the result of the manipulation of societal consumption by the corporate elite and its

[1] It is worth underlining that the category *poor* is presented unconnected with any class linkage. The fact that all poor people are, by association, employment or unemployment, members of the working class is dismissed, since the category of *working class* has assumedly disappeared altogether.

[2] In this article, the American terms "conservative" and "liberal" will be used interchangeably with the European term "bourgeois." Conservative, liberal or bourgeois positions are those positions that do not question but rather build upon the basic assumptions of capitalism.

different components, including the medical and other professions and bureaucracies.

In summary, then, according to the majority of conservative and liberal social analysts, and including large sectors of left-wing writers as well, social class has lost its importance as a category of social analysis that would explain not only the nature of Western societies but also the different patterns of production and consumption within them. As a result of that belief, these analysts have concluded that past class inequalities in the distribution and consumption of resources have been superseded by persisting or newly created inequalities such as those of age, sex, and regional imbalance.[3]

Middle Class-Mass Society, Political Power, and the State: An Analysis of Theories

A most important consequence of the prevalent belief that we are a middle class society—or in its newer version, that we are a mass society— is the idea that class struggle has been superseded. Instead, it is assumed that conflict and struggle exist not among classes—passé social categories—but among groups and elites. And it is believed that the nature and outcome of those conflicts—and not of class struggle—explain the nature and content of Western developed societies, including the composition and distribution of societal resources such as medical resources. Reflecting this set of beliefs are two prevalent bodies of doctrine that, in most political sociology and political economy literature, aim at explaining the distribution of political power in Western societies. One includes the different variations of those paradigms that have usually been referred to as the theories of pluralistic countervailing power, while the other group encompasses those theories that have come to be known as the power elite paradigms. Because of the frequency with which both groups of theories appear in the analysis of our society and its sectors, including the medical care sector, let me summarize them here.

[3]The assumption that Cochrane (reference 1), for example, makes in dismissing class inequalities and in their stead focusing on age and regional ones, is that age and regional differences are independent from and unrelated to class differences. This assumption, however, is an erroneous one. For example, if we analyze the interregional differences in availability of human health resources in the NHS, we see that those regions with higher percentages of the working class (and primarily of the low-income strata within it) are also the ones with lower availability of resources. See reference 13 for a discussion of regional disparities in health services.

Countervailing Pluralist Theories of Power

According to these theories, our societies have neither dominant classes nor dominant groups or elites. Rather, there exist competing blocs of interests, with no one having a dominant control over the state,[4] which is assumed to be an independent entity. In the words of one proponent of this theory:

> Government becomes more or less another group or interest in cooperation, competition, and negotiation with the private individual or groups (17).

In such explanations of our societies (see, for example, references 13 and 14), power is thought to be diffuse, with different competing blocs balancing each other and themselves, and with no particular group or interest being able to weigh too heavily upon the state. It is furthermore believed that it is this very competition among interests, supervised and arbitrated by the state, which provides the prime guarantee against the concentration of that power. A system is thus created that offers the possibility for all active and legitimate groups in the population to make themselves heard at any crucial stage in the decision-making process (18). And this "being heard" takes place primarily through a parliamentarian system in which a plurality of ideas are openly exchanged, complementary to the free allocation of resources that occurs in the marketplace and following, for the most part, the rules of laissez-faire. It is, of course, recognized that the system is far from perfect. But, in any case, those societies are considered to have already achieved a model of democracy in light of which the notion of "ruling class" or even "power elite" is ludicrous, completely irrelevant, and of concern only to ideologues.

The main weakness of such paradigms, however, is not so much their postulate that competition exists, but more importantly, their unmindfulness that such competition is continuously and consistently skewed in favor of some groups and against others. As the power elite theorists have empirically shown, the different organs of the state are heavily influenced and in some instances dominated by specific power groups. In that

---

[4] In the term "state," I include the executive and legislative branches of government as well as the state apparatus, i.e. the administrative bureaucracy, the judiciary, the army and the police. Also, it is important to clarify that I consider the state to be far more than the mere aggregate of those institutions. Rather, it includes the set of relationships between and among those institutions and with other ones that it guides and directs (such as the medical institutions). These relationships are aimed, as I will show later on in this article, at perpetuating and reproducing the system of production and its concomitant class relations. To understand the nature of the state in Western societies, three excellent volumes are references 14, 15 and 16.

respect, the pluralist's failure to recognize the consistent dominance of our state organs by specific groups is certainly not shared by the majority of the U.S. population, who believe, for example, that both political parties are in favor of big business and that America's major corporations dominate and determine the behavior of our public officials and of the different branches of the state (19).

Power Elite Theories of Political Power

The limited value of the pluralist theories in terms of explaining our political realities accounts for the increased development of analytical paradigms such as the power elite theories, which have eclipsed much of the prominence of the pluralistic explanations. According to these newer paradigms, the postulated pluralism applies only to a very limited segment within our societies, i.e. a small number of elite groups which essentially dominate the different branches of the state.

Considerable variation exists among power elite theorists, but all of them use a similar conceptualization and methodology. Their most frequent method of analysis includes, first, identification of the groups or elites that play a dominant role in the different sectors of the state; second, analysis of how that power is exercised and through which mechanisms of state intervention; and third, description of the nature of the benefits those groups obtain as a result of their intervention. This method of analysis has been especially prevalent in the study of the medical care sector (20), where the various actors, i.e. hospitals, universities, insurance companies, physicians, etc. are seen as competing power groups in their quest for dominance of and/or influence in the different agencies of the state. According to this analysis, the campagne de bataille is the control of knowledge, licensure, instruments of care, funds, etc. It is worth underlining that the contribution of these authors to the understanding of our sector has not been small. Quite to the contrary, they have provided extremely valuable empirical information for the analysis of the health sector in Western societies. However, their focus on the health sector together with their seeming unawareness of social class, has seriously limited the explanatory value of their theories. Indeed, as I have indicated in earlier articles, in order to understand the behavior and dynamics of the actors in the health sector, we have to understand their positions within the overall economic and political scheme of our societies, i.e. their class positions. In this respect, the main limitation of the power elite theories is their failure to recognize that those elites are in reality segments of a dominant class and that when they are considered in a systemic and not just a sectorial fashion, they are found to possess a high degree of cohesion and solidarity, with common interests and common purposes far transcending their specific differences and disagreements. Consequently, those authors do not include in their analysis the non-actors and the non-decisions which may be far more important than the visible and intervening actors and the studied actual decisions. In other words, the competitive (as the pluralist theorists believe) or not-so-competitive (as the power elite theorists postulate) conflict among power groups or elites in Western societies for dominance and even control of the organs of the state takes place within a set of class relations and within a well-defined capitalist structure whose maintenance and reproduction is the primary role of the state, the subject of that competition. This state role establishes a set of constraints (which I will detail later) in that competition that are of paramount importance in understanding the nature of the conflict and of the system. And again, in that competition among groups and elites, the non-actors and non-decisions are as important as, if not more important than, the actors and decisions. In fact, both non-decisions and decisions respond to the dynamics of the Western societies—societies that I will redefine as capitalist societies and that have a rationality of their own (21).

A further weakness of the power elite theories—a weakness that the structuralist theories, to be described later on, attempt to remedy—is that there is a very real risk that the nature of the system will be defined as one of conflict resolution among different groups of actors and individuals whose *behavior* and *motivation* determine the nature of the conflict. In that respect, such analysis leads to viewing personalities and their motivations as the predominant forces in those conflicts (22).

A new variation of these power elite interpretations appears in the writings of authors who define the nature of our societies and the sectors within them as the result of the ideological manipulation of our populations by the bureaucracies (including the professional bureaucracies), which are assumed to have replaced the capitalist class as the main agencies of oppression. According to these theories of bureaucratic and professional control, the process of industrialization has reshaped the nature of our societies in such a way that power, assumed to be divorced from ownership of capital, has passed from the owners of capital—the capitalists—to the managers of that capital, and from there to the technocrats—those who have the skills and knowledge needed to operate the major social edifices of industrialism, the bureaucracies. The new elite, then, are the bureaucrats, who have supplanted the capitalists. In medicine, for example, Illich (23), one of the main proponents of this theory, assumes that the nature of medicine and medical care is very much the result of the manipulation of medical resources (including the ideology of medicine) by the medical bureaucracy, which, in order to perpetuate its power, has created an addiction to medicine that legitimizes the control over the population by the medical profession. More recently, powerful voices in international agencies have responded sympathetically to that interpretation (24). Since I have discussed this theory and its political implications elsewhere (25), I do not intend to repeat here what I consider to be its main conceptual, methodological and political weaknesses, except to indicate my belief that while the medical profession is very much part of the problem, it is not *the* problem. Indeed, a historical, empirical, and political analysis of the health sector indicates that (a) the most predominant force in determining the nature of medicine and the resulting iatrogeneses and dependencies has been not the medical profession, but the capitalist system and the capitalist class; (b) for the most part, medical professionals are the administrators and not the creators of these dependencies; and (c) this interpretation of bureaucratic and professional power and control leads to a strategy that ultimately strengthens the ideological construct of capitalism.

Regarding the first two points, Susser (26) has convincingly shown that the way medical problems are defined and the way strategies for solving them are implemented is in response to the needs of society as perceived and defined by the powerful. And this process of continuous redefinition takes place in spite of the medical profession's resistance to those changes. On a scale of determinants, the medical profession's influence is secondary to a higher hierarchical level of dominance. It is because of their unawareness of this gradient of determinants and their focus instead on the medical profession that these authors' strategy of anti-medicine and self-care is easily co-optable. Indeed, the solutions of self-reliance, self-care, and the independence and autonomy of the individual suggested by them assume that the individual is ultimately responsible for his or her own health. And it is because this interpretation does not conflict with the tenets of the capitalist system (e.g. individualism) that we frequently find rebellious authors such as Illich with strange bedfellows like President Ford. Recall, for example, the great stress in Ford's recent State of the Union message on self-care, health education and changes in life style as the primary health strategy of a profoundly conservative administration. In summary, these authors, conservatives and rebels alike, see changes in the individual and not changes in the system of class relations and its system of production as the primary solution. Their main weakness, of course, is their unawareness of the rationale and requirements of the capitalist system, which is itself the primary creator of dependencies and determines the nature of sickness and its perpetuation in our societies.

A Critique of Some Marxist Theories of Political Power and of the State

The limitations of the pluralist and power elite theories in explaining our continuously and increasingly "in-crisis" societies, as well as the overall expansion of socialist movements all over the world, have led to the appearance of new analyses that establish a profound divergence from the earlier theories in their recognition of the nature and structure of capitalism as the main explanatory "variable" for understanding what is going on in our societies and sectors. All of them take Marx (not Weber, as the previous theories did) as their point of departure. Because of the great importance of these theories, let me outline them according to three subgroups that I define, perhaps somewhat arbitrarily, as (a) economic determinist, (b) structural determinist, and (c) corporate statist.

Economic Determinism

Miliband (27), Poulantzas (28) and others include in the first group those theorists who assume that whatever happens or does not happen in political life depends primarily and exclusively on what is going on at the economic level of society. In other words, the laws of economic development linearly and mechanistically determine the laws of political and social development, i.e. the economic needs of capitalism determine the nature of our political systems. Capitalism, once reduced to its economic dimensions, appears as a system that is evolving unavoidably and fatalistically according to its internal economic laws. In this scheme, the role of state intervention is seen primarily as that of smoothing out any contradictions and bottlenecks that might handicap the evolution of the economic mode of production. This economic determinism finds two expressions in the interpretation of the medical sector in Western developed societies. One version, prevalent in the literature of political economy, perceives changes in the nature, form, and distribution of resources in the medical sector as being exclusively determined by the economic needs of the capitalist system. The other version maintains that the changes in the mode of production in medicine reflect the changes in the mode of production of capitalism, i.e. from petty commodity production (cottage industry) to large-scale commodity production (monopoly capital). In these theories, there is the belief that the organizational evolution of medicine (from cottage medicine to corporate medicine) is exclusively determined by the changes in the mode of production of medicine, which follow and replicate the different stages of the economic development of capitalism.

The great merit of these contributions has been their rediscovery of the economic nature and function of the health sector, representing a break with the prevalent Hegelian and idealistic interpretations that saw the evolution of medicine as a result of personalities and values, without realizing the purpose of those values within the rationality of the economic system. The limitations of these contributions, however, are in viewing history as a fatalistic and deterministic process and not, as Marx saw it, as a dialectical one (29). Indeed, to indicate the importance and even primacy of the economic base does not imply the reduction of history to its economic laws of motion. There are other factors and levels such as politics, religion, medicine, etc. that continuously interact with the economic base as well as among themselves and thus contribute to the formation of history. As Engels indicated:

> Political, religious, juridical, philosophical, literary, artistic, etc. [and I would add medical] development is based on economic development. But all these react upon one another and also upon the economic bases. It is not that the economic situation is *cause, solely active,* while everything else is only passive effect. There is, rather, interaction on the basis of economic necessity, which *ultimately* always asserts itself (30).

Let me underline here that by criticizing the economic determinists, I do not mean to detract from the extremely important and primary role that the analysis of the economic base has in understanding the realm of the possible in our societies. As Marx indicated:

> Men make their own history, but they do not make it just as they please; they do not make it under circumstances chosen by themselves but under circumstances directly encountered, given, and transmitted from the past (31).

And among those circumstances, the economic ones are of primary importance. Consequently, I have stressed elsewhere (32) the great need to study the material bases of history in order to understand the evolution of medicine in any society. In that respect, I am an historical materialist and proud of it. My criticism of the economic determinists should be read primarily as a criticism of their seeming unmindfulness to the importance of other factors besides economics in determining why changes in capitalism and its medicine take place and take the form that they do.

Structural Determinism

I define structural determinists as those theorists who while aware of the limitations of economic determinism, nonetheless believe that there are objective laws of motion in capitalism that *wholly* determine how classes and their substrata operate. Heavily influenced by Althusser (33), Godelier (34), Poulantzas (35) and other French structuralists, those theorists assume that who is in government, for example, or what groups dominate what state boards, is not important since the laws of the system (its objective relations) are so constraining that intergroup conflicts and relations are of little consequence, and the structure of the capitalist system explains and/or constrains everything (36). Here, we find ourselves at the other extreme from the power elite theoreticians. Indeed, while the power elite analysts fail to recognize the importance of the structure of capitalism in their analysis of the competition between elites, the structural determinists believe that structure and the set of objective relations determined by it explain everything. At the highest level of abstraction, the latter position leads to the statement that the structure of the capitalist system is the source of all our problems. But this understanding can yield little unless those categories, structures and relations are disaggregated and their political nature and implications are verified empirically. In other words, there is no capitalism without a capitalist class; and that class is composed of different segments or fractions that interact dialectically. The specific form that capitalism takes depends[5] on the nature of the class struggle[5] and of the internecine

---

[5] By class struggle is meant the realization of the economic, political and social conflict among social classes and primarily between the capitalist class and the working class. According to bourgeois theory, there is no intrinsic conflict between Capital and Labor. Rather, they are supposed to complement each other. According to Marxist theory, to which I subscribe, there is an intrinsic conflict between both. The advantage of one presupposes the disadvantage of the other. Actually, not only Marxists, but leading representatives of Capital have subscribed to this paradigm. None other than Gates (37), the closest advisor to J.D. Rockefeller, indicated that "the plank between Capital and Labor is stiff. If labor goes up, capital comes down; if capital goes up, labor goes down. There are no two ways about it, it is impossible, utterly impossible, unthinkable, unimaginable that labor as a whole can have increase of wages except capital as a whole shall have a decrease of interest and rent." And this paradigm is verified by data representing the distribution of national income, i.e. when income to labor increases, income to capital declines, and vice versa (38).

struggles among segments within the capitalist class. Actually, not only does the structure of capitalism condition the class struggle, but more importantly and conversely, the class struggle and the conflict between factions within the capitalist class condition and determine the structure of capitalism.[6] Not to be aware of the latter aspect might lead, as Miliband rightly indicates, to the conclusion that there are no differences between a state ruled by fascists and one ruled by social democrats, since both are capitalist systems.

Corporate Statism

Another body of theory is that of corporate statism, which views the state as the direct instrument of the capitalist class or of one of its components, the corporate class (42). Here, Marx and Engels' statement that "the modern state is but a committee for managing the common affairs of the whole bourgeoisie" (43) is taken to mean that the state not only acts on behalf of, but at the behest of, the capitalist class. In that interpretation, the state and the capitalist class (or a segment within it, the corporate class) are in a symbiotic relationship, i.e. the one is the other. It is interesting to note that this theory of the corporate state, as Gough has pointed out, is especially prevalent today in U.S. Marxist literature because, among other political items, a Rockefeller is the vice-president of the country, and the degree of personal penetration by corporate groups of the organs of the state is very high indeed (44). Thus, there is considerable temptation to believe that the state acts not only on behalf of, but also at the behest of, the capitalist class and that the evolution of all sectors, including the health sector, is the result of manipulation of the agencies of the state by different segments of the capitalist class and its dependent upper-middle class, including the professions. Similar analyses and interpretations appear in the U.K., France, and Germany, particularly (although not exclusively) when conservative governments are in power.

The limitation of these theories is their seeming unawareness that there is a clear distinction between "on behalf of" and "at the behest of." In fact, the state, to better serve the capitalist class, needs to be autonomous (but not, as I will explain later, independent). And the degree of that autonomy depends primarily on the level and form of class struggle in a given society, including, for example, the existence of a political party based on and supported by the working class. Indeed, the absence of a political arm of American labor has made Capital subject to

[6] For an interesting debate on this point, see references 39–41.

far fewer restrictions in the U.S. than it has been in Britain or in Continental Europe, for example. And this has led to the predominance of members of the capitalist class in the different organs of the state, including its executive and legislative branches. But that predominance, empirically shown in all sectors of the state, is not tantamount to direct control. And the failure to recognize this fact may lead to the dismissal of the state as a proper champ de bataille, i.e. to a rejection of participation in the parliamentary system to advance working class-based programs.

SECTION II:

THE ROLE, NATURE, CHARACTERISTICS AND
MODE OF STATE INTERVENTION

The Role of State Intervention

Having made a critique of the prevalent interpretations of political power and of the state, let me now outline my own interpretation of the state, both within and outside the health sector, touching on its main areas that doubtless will require further exposition, detail, and empirical verification in the subsequent stages of development of this work.

And the first postulate I would make is that the state in our societies is the configuration of public institutions and their relationships whose primary role is the reproduction of an economic system based on private ownership of the means of production, i.e. the capitalist economy. Let me clarify here that I am aware, of course, of the prevalent mythology that due to the dramatic expansion of the public sector since World War II (assumedly because of the Keynesian revolution), our economies are no longer capitalist but mixed economies. Empirical information shows, however, that in none of the so-called mixed economy countries does the state own more than a subsidiary and complementary part of the means of production. And it is because of this that, as Miliband correctly points out, to speak of mixed economies in this context is "to attribute a special and quite misleading meaning to the notion of mixture" (45). We do indeed have a capitalist system with a capitalist class whose power derives from its ownership and control over the means of production. And a primary role of the state is to establish the conditions for the survival and flourishing of that economic system. For example, both Labour and Conservative governments in the United Kingdom and Democratic and Republican administrations in the United States have indicated that their primary role and concern is the "health" of the economy, with everything else being conditional on its survival and improvement. To have social services or to expand their benefits depends on having a "healthy" economy. The assumption that is made in all these cases, of course, is that the welfare of the people depends, first and foremost, on the welfare of the economy. But what is meant by the economy is the capitalist economy in which the capitalist class rules.

How does the state establish the conditions for the economy to operate? In many different ways, the most important of which are the following:

- *The development of what is usually referred to as the infrastructure of production,* i.e. the development of those goods and services that are the preconditions for the functioning of the capitalist system—goods and services that are essential as
  - (a) *technical* preconditions for the actual process of production (e.g. roads, railways, environmental and sanitation services, postal service, etc.);
  - (b) *social* preconditions of this same process (e.g. law and order, a stable currency system, etc.); and
  - (c) conditions for the *reproduction of labor* (e.g. education and some preventive health services).

  All of these goods and services have the characteristic that for only one individual or corporation to buy them would be either too costly or too risky, in the sense that making a profit would be uncertain or the possibilities of monopolizing their use would be very limited (46).

- *The defense of the capitalist system* through
  - (a) The actual delivery of goods and services in response to different pressures mediated in the political process, of which the most important pressures are those generated by the class struggle. That provision of services is aimed (not always successfully) at increasing the level of cohesion among classes and groups in a society and avoiding its disruption. Thus, social legislation (such as social security, for example) has historically been implemented at moments of labor unrest (47). And as Balfour indicated in 1895, "Social legislation is not merely to be distinguished from Socialist legislation, but it is its most direct opposite and its most effective antidote" (48).
  - (b) The development and/or maintenance of the value-generating institutions such as the media, academia, and others which sustain a system of values that, while appearing natural, universal or commonsensical, are actually the values (e.g.

individualism and competitiveness) most convenient to the
survival of the economic system. And included in this value
system as its societal and ethical pillar is the primacy of the
private sector and profit-making. Consequently, all activities
that make a profit should be left to the private sector and
conversely, all activities should be geared, to the highest degree
possible, to the generation of profit. The public sector should
intervene only when the private activity is too costly or too risky
or, in the penultimate hour, when it has failed.

- *The control over physical force,* to be used against internal and
external threats against the system.

It is important to note that for the state to be able to establish the
first two conditions, it must be perceived, at least by the majority of the
population, as being neutral, above classes, and serving common
interests. In that respect, its claims to put the state of the economy first are
legitimized as necessary for the benefit of everyone in society. Calls to
austerity and sacrifice are, in theory, calls for all, since we are all in the
same boat, i.e. the capitalist economy. As Offe has recently indicated,
"The existence of a capitalist state presupposes the systematic denial of its
nature as a capitalist state" (49). It is when the legitimation disintegrates
and the supposedly classless nature of the state is being questioned that
the state resorts to physical force, the third condition.

What Defines a State as Capitalist?

The capitalist character of the state is attributable not to its being the state
of the capitalist class (or its corporate component, as some corporate
statists postulate) but, far more importantly, to the fact that the state's
primary role is to defend, support, and encourage the capitalist economy,
upon whose health (or lack of it) everything else is assumed to depend.
Therefore, what establishes governments as capitalist is not so much that
members of the capitalist class predominate in them (50), but, most
importantly,

   (a)   that they give primacy not to the interests of specific capitalist
         groups, but to the interests of the capitalist economy as a whole,
         whose sanctity is considered to be above the interests of specific
         groups or classes; and
   (b)   that when a conflict appears between what are considered to be
         the needs of the economy and other needs such as an increase in

the satisfaction of human needs, the former takes priority over the latter. Present day examples are the dramatic cuts in allocations for social services in both Wilson's and Ford's 1977 fiscal budgets. In both cases, the rationale for the cuts is that they are perceived as needed to save the troubled economies of the U.K. (51) and of the U.S. (52).

In summary, to see these policies as a result of malevolence of individuals or the manipulation of government by certain economic groups is, in my opinion, both limited and erroneous. Such policies respond to the need perceived by those governments that the economy, to whose health we are all supposedly tied, has to be straightened out before "we can think of others matters." And it is this behavior, and not the specific motivation of individuals or manipulation by groups, which establishes those policies as capitalist policies. The fact that the policies required to save the capitalist system are sometimes made against the interests of specific capitalist groups (as during the New Deal) does not make them any less capitalistic. Actually, the state is better able to represent the interests of the capitalist class as a whole when it can be politically autonomous from specific short or even long term economic interests or particular fractions of that class.

The Characteristics of the Capitalist State

Having explained why states in Western developed societies are capitalist states, and the necessity of relative autonomy of the state from the capitalist class, let me now focus on the mechanisms which establish the dominance of that class over the state. These mechanisms are (a) the dependence of the state on the successful development of the capitalist economies, (b) the class origins of the top members of the organs of the state, (c) the ideology of the state, and (d) the structure of the state, with the principle of separation of powers. Due to the importance of each, let us analyze them in more detail.

The Dependency of the State on the Successful Development of the Capitalist Economies

The size and scope of state activities depend heavily on the successful development of the economy. State activities are funded through revenues collected via taxes on wages and profits realized in the economy, and through credit, increasing the national debt. And the mass of wages, profits and credit depend very much on the state of "health" of the economy (53). When the latter suffers, the former shrinks. Consequently, it is of paramount importance for the expansion of the state that the process of capital accumulation—the axle that keeps the economy moving—takes place in as unobstructed and smooth a way as is politically possible, since state resources depend on that capital accumulation. As Offe has indicated, "accumulation . . . acts as the most powerful constraint criterion, but not necessarily as the determinant of content, of the policy-making process" (54). This dependency of state activities and resources on the overall health of the economy is clearly shown in the present fiscal crises of the state. Let us consider, for instance, how social security and large numbers of health programs are affected by the state of the economy. The funding of both types of programs is very seriously handicapped in the present economic crunch, since that crunch means less revenue into the Treasury's coffers from which come the money to pay for them. And this scarcity of revenue is felt most intensely precisely at a time when the need for expansion of those programs is becoming more acute since, due to the poor state of the economy, there is more unemployment, earlier retirement, increased sickness, etc. In other words, it is precisely when the state needs to provide those services to show that it works and can take care of people when necessary that it can least afford to do so, since capital is needed to save the economy and cannot be diverted into social expenditures. Thus the predicament is that the time when the state needs to appear most classless, for purposes of legitimation, is the very time when its class nature appears most clearly.

It is important to stress here that this dependency of the state and its apparatus on the "health" of the economy is of paramount importance to understanding not only national but also international governmental policies. Indeed, the integration and increasing interdependence of their economies make nation states more vulnerable and dependent than ever before on the "health" of the world capitalist system. An example of this dependency of state policies on international economic demands is the reported pressure that administrators of the Marshall Plan brought to bear on successive British governments to reduce the size of the public sector in the U.K., including limiting NHS expenditures. Indeed, Marshall Plan aid was made conditional on increasing military expenditures, liberalizing trade, and cutting social programs, including housing, health, and education (55). The development of the latter—social programs—was subordinated and made conditional to the successful implementation of the former—the liberalization of trade and expansion of military expenditures.

The Class Origin of the Top Members
of the Organs of the State

The class origin of the top members of the state organs has been well documented by, among others, Domhoff (56) in the U.S. and Miliband (57) in the U.K. Similarly, Tudor Hart (58) in Britain and I (59) in the U.S. have shown the pattern of class dominance in the main organs of the medical care sectors in both societies. Here again, it is important to stress that what determines the class composition of the state is the class nature of our societies and vice versa, i.e. what imparts a capitalist character to the state is its function, not its composition.[7] In a class society it is just "natural" that those in positions of power belong, for the most part, to the capitalist class, either by origin, association, or the sharing of beliefs. As Mandel has indicated, "The capitalist state machine . . . possesses a hierarchical organization correspondent to the order of the capitalist society itself" (60).

Here, let me add a note that I believe to be of great importance, and that concerns the key significance of the composition and ideology of the state. A recent debate between Poulantzas and Miliband (61) has centered on the importance of that composition in defining, explaining, and understanding the nature of the state. Poulantzas believes that what establishes a state as capitalist is its function, as mentioned before, and not its composition. I fully agree with this (and so, for that matter, does Miliband). But Poulantzas goes still further, maintaining that even if all of the members of the state, including its apparatus, were not members of the capitalist class by origin, i.e. if they were working class, that state would still be capitalist—a position which I find linear, non-dialectical, deterministic, and most un-Marxian. Indeed, the high degree of abstraction and generalization in which French structuralists indulge and their disregard for empirical verification leads them to miss the point, i.e. in not one of the capitalist societies (including the assumedly socialist society of Sweden) do members of the working class have more than a minimal role in the top corridors of the state and its apparatus. For example, the number of workers' sons and daughters in the top political echelons in Sweden in 1961 was less than 9 per cent (62). And as long as these societies are capitalist, those at the top of the state will be members of the capitalist class. Moreover, because of their failure to analyze the actual composition of the state and its meaning in policy formulation, the French structuralists and other adherents to this approach run the risk of

[7]The function is what determines the class position; the origin is what determines the class situation. See reference 16 for further explanation.

blurring the distinction between a state run by fascists and one run by social democrats, since both are capitalist. Let me add a personal note here. As one who has lived under both fascist and social democratic regimes, I can testify that there were plenty of differences, not only for me, but more importantly, for the working class. It is because of this difference, for example, that the major underground Marxist parties in Spain are supporting the reestablishment of bourgeois democracy (63). Actually, the real point of the story about bourgeois democracy is not that it is irrelevant, but rather that it is dramatically insufficient.

Reflecting the class nature and class position of the state and its apparatus, we find that the top echelons of the civil service share an ideology that gives that apparatus an internal cohesiveness and logic of its own. And that ideology is the one of the capitalist class. It is the glue that keeps the pieces together, and another mechanism through which the dominance of the capitalist class over the state becomes established. Indeed, "success" in the civil service is related not so much to competence but primarily to the degree to which performance conforms to the tenets of those in power. It is utterly inconceivable, for example, that a person either rejecting or resisting the existing social order and its norms of thought and action could reach the top of the state apparatus. Indeed:

> Convinced and active pacifists do not usually become generals, and it is absolutely certain that they do not become Chiefs of General Staff. To imagine that the bourgeois state apparatus could be used for a socialist transformation of capitalist society is as illusory as to suppose that an army could be dissolved with the aid of "pacifist generals" (64).

Similarly, it would be unimaginable that the Secretary of HEW in the United States or the top senior medical officer in Britain would believe in a classless society, with workers and community control of the health institutions.

In summary, there is a set of beliefs that members of the state apparatus must hold. One example is the belief required of them—and, for the most part, gladly held—regarding the primacy of the private sector. In fact, some of the strongest opponents of public ownership are individuals serving the state apparatus. See, for example, the recent declarations by the New York City Health Commissioner in support of the absorption of the New York municipal hospitals by the voluntary private ones (65). Needless to say, the frequent turnover and exchange of job opportunities between the public and private sectors, with public officials waiting for beneficial retirement in the private sector after they leave public service, further contributes to what is already a natural condition and consequence of the internal logic of the system.

I am aware, of course, of the argument that those civil servants are just reflecting the overall values of the society, and also that, for the most part, they are above specific economic or class interests. Indeed, as I indicated earlier, this appearance of being above class interests is of paramount importance to legitimizing both their conduct and the state apparatus. But empirical evidence shows that, for the most part, their ideas are the ideas of the powerful in society. And among these ideas, an important one is the primacy of the private sector and the need for strengthening the capitalist system, usually expressed in terms of "strengthening the economy." And the same applies, incidentally, to the series of advisory and consultant bodies set up by the state apparatus. Many studies have shown the predominance of members who uphold bourgeois positions in most advisory, policy-making bodies in the branches of the state. In the health sector, for example, we can see that the large majority of members of the present National Health Planning Council appointed by the Secretary of HEW are well known believers in the sanctity of the private sector. In fact, one of the leading forces on that council (assumed to be the main federal health planning advisory body) is an individual usually referred to as the Milton Friedman of the health sector, and whose main ideological distinction is his defense of and support for the reintegration of the private market forces in the medical care sector (66). "Free marketeers" in command of the top health planning advisory body! Similarly, out of nearly 100 members of the special advisory board on national health insurance set up by the U.S. Congress, very few are publicly known advocates or supporters either of any form of national health service or of workers' control in the health sector (67). And this is so despite the fact that 22 per cent of the U.S. citizenry have declared their support for a completely federally financed and owned health system (68), and 62 per cent expressed the need for workers' control (69). Needless to say, in order to serve the legitimation function I alluded to before, all those advisory bodies need to be presented as being balanced, professional, and for the most part, absent of "ideologues" and most certainly absent of class interest.

The Structure of the State and the Separation of Powers

A final and most important determinant of class power in capitalist societies is inherent in the structure of the state itself and its principle of

separation of powers, wherein the bodies responsible for the implementation of policies are separate from the bodies responsible for deciding and
formulating those policies. This decision making and formulation, however, takes place indirectly—by supposed representatives of the population seated in the executive and legislative branches of government—and
not directly by the population itself. Thus, Western democracies are
indirect democracies and, we may add, incomplete democracies. Indeed,
due to the skewed nature of political debate, political parties which
question the basic assumptions of the capitalist system are systematically
hindered from participating in the electoral system and seriously
handicapped from presenting their views in the marketplace of ideas, to
the advantage of those parties which do accept the system.

Moreover, the indirect character of Western democracies is being
increasingly strengthened by the remarkable shift of the power of political
decision making from the legislative to the executive branch of
government and to the central administrative machinery, a shift which
has left an indelible imprint on most Western parliamentarian and
congressional systems. And this shift of power is not independent of nor
unrelated to the shift of the capitalist mode of production from
competitive to monopolistic. Indeed, the increasing concentration of state
policy within the executive branch and the central administration
corresponds not so much to the requirements of the increasingly complex
post-industrial societies, but rather to the increased centralization of
economic power and its dominance over both the executive and
administrative branches of government. Actually, I would postulate that
the growing centralization of economic and management policies in the
NHS (with the 1974 reorganization) and of health planning in the U.S.
(reflected in the National Health Planning Act of 1975),[8] are a response to
pressures on the state organs by the monopolistic segments in both
societies to do something about the "mess" in the health and social sectors
(70). Not infrequently, this process of centralization and increased
bureaucratization further strengthens the tendency inherent in the
internal rationale of the capitalist system to separate the governors from
the governed and the administrators from those administered or, as Lenin
indicated, to separate the State from Society (71).

Politics in bourgeois democracies, therefore, takes place in the realm
of the politicians—the experts in the art of politicking—and not in
people's everyday lives. As a recent powerful international commission on

[8]That centralization takes place by the central government's appointment of ad hoc bodies
ultimately accountable to it, and the subsequent bypassing of state and local authorities.

the study of Western democracies indicated, Western democracies work best when the citizenry is passive and somewhat apathetic, and when its input into the political process takes place only through a limited electoral system (72). Thus, the implied, and I might add, actual function of the electoral system is to legitimize the political process rather than to secure the people's input in their own governance. In consequence, as Wolfe has recently indicated, the electoral aim is the replication of a political institution "which claims primary responsibility for reproducing alienated politics, that is, for maintaining a political system based upon the extraction and imposition of power from people" (73). Not surprisingly then, and as part of the increased consciousness of the population and the intensification of class struggle, that process of legitimization is quickly losing its validity. In fact, a primary problem in Western societies, and one documented by numerous recent opinion polls, is the alienation of increased masses of the population (in the case of the U.S., the majority) from the political system. And that disenchantment with the system of government has been an increasing process, not a declining one. According to the University of Michigan's Survey Research Data, there was a growing decline of public trust in government between 1964 and 1970 and an equally sharp rise in the feeling that government is run only by and for the rich (74).

The Characteristics and Consequences of State Intervention in the Health Sector

Having explained the characteristics of the state intervention in capitalist societies, let me now focus on the specific characteristics of capitalist state intervention in the health sector. But first, let me clarify that the health sector is increasingly part of the state. This occurs because (a) the production and allocation of health resources are perceived in most Western capitalist societies as public responsibilities, where the chartering of resources and services has to be approved by the public sector; (b) training, research and the delivery of services are increasingly financed from public funds; and (c) the ideology and organization of medicine build upon and strengthen the replication of class relations in our society, thus reinforcing the capitalist system. In that respect, the ideology of the capitalist system, guaranteed by the nature of the state intervention, is embodied in the ideology of medicine and in the medical institutions themselves. Indeed, as Gramsci (75) has indicated, the state directs and involves itself in most spheres of political, social and economic life, and the ideological influence of the state apparatus far transcends the sector that we usually refer to as the public sector. And medicine is very much a part of it, regardless of whether those medical institutions are, legally speaking, private or public. Thus, in the Gramscian sense, I am including in the public sector all those institutions affected by the state apparatus, i.e. not only medicine, but also academia, the media, etc.

The Reproduction of Class Structure

Within the health sector, the state replicates the class hierarchy that characterizes capitalist societies. Accordingly, the distribution of functions and responsibilities within the health labor force follows class, sex, and racial lines with, for example, physicians being primarily uppermiddle class white males; nurses, lower-middle or working class females; and auxiliary health workers, females of working class backgrounds. And as I have shown elsewhere (76), both the distribution of skills and knowledge and the control of technology are aimed at strengthening the class relations within the health sector. To assume, as Illich and others do, that control over technology is what gives the medical profession its power is to be unhistorical and unempirical. A study of underlying causes shows that the hierarchy was already there, and that technology strengthened it, not vice versa. Needless to say, both the hierarchy and technology strengthen each other in a dialectical fashion, i.e. each one has influence on the other. But in that dialectical relationship, hierarchy based on class comes first and takes precedence over the other (77).

The Reproduction of Bourgeois Ideology

Moreover, state intervention replicates the ideology of medicine which complements, rather than conflicts, with the ideology of capitalism, i.e. liberalism and individualism. And this ideology of medicine takes two forms that relate dialectically not only with each other, but also with the ideology of capitalism, which subsumes the ideology of medicine. One form is the mechanistic conception of medicine, in which it is assumed that disease is the imbalance of the components of the machine-like body. As McKeown has eloquently presented it, the most prevalent approach to medicine, Flexnerianism, has been (and still is) that "a living organism could be regarded as a machine which might be taken apart and reassembled if its structure and functions were fully understood" (78). And the second form, which derives from the first, is that the cause of disease is primarily individual, and thus the therapeutic response to it is individually oriented. Increasing historical evidence suggests that the victory of Flexnerianism in U.S. medicine paralleled the increasing influence of corporate America on the state. Similarly, the vision of scientific medicine in Europe in the late nineteenth century represented a victory of the individualistic-mechanistic view over the environmentalist-structuralist one (advocated by the revolutionary Virchow), replicating in the health sector the conflict between Weberian and Marxist interpretations of reality.

At a time when most disease was socially determined due to the conditions of nascent capitalism (79), an ideology that saw the "fault" of disease as lying with the individual and that emphasized the individual therapeutic response clearly absolved the economic and political environment from the responsibility for disease and channeled potential response and rebellion against that environment to an individual, and thus less threatening level. The ideology of medicine was the individualization of a collective causality that by its very nature would have required a collective answer.

That Flexnerian medicine today serves a similarly apologist function is clear to see. Let us analyze, for example, three major health problems in today's capitalist societies: (a) alienation of the individual in society, which is responsible for a majority of the psychosomatic conditions seen in medical practice and is largely due to the lack of control felt by our citizenry over their own work and over societal institutions (80); (b) occupational diseases, the etiology of which is very much the result of control of the labor process by capital and not by labor, with profit making taking priority over job safety and workers' satisfaction; and (c) cancer, determined in its overwhelming majority of cases by environmental conditions, with individuals living in industrial working class neighborhoods facing a much greater risk of dying of cancer than those who live in residential areas.

These are just three examples of the economic and political etiology of disease, and this aspect is as apparent today as when our diseases were predominantly infectious ones. But, and as one would expect, the response of the powerful in society is either to deny or to obscure that reality. Instead, the cause of the problem is perceived as individual, and the nature of intervention is individually oriented (health education in prevention and clinical medicine in cure). Consequently, one of today's most active state policies at the central governmental level in most Western capitalist countries is to encourage and stimulate those health programs, such as health education, that are aimed at bringing about

changes in the individual but not in the economic or political environment (81).

It is interesting to note that while much of the disease affecting the
working class in Engels' time was supposedly due to the poor moral fiber
of the workers and their families, today the poor health conditions of that
class and of the majority of the population are assumed to be due to their
lack of concern for their own health and their poor health education. In
both cases, the solution to our public's lack of health is *individual*
prevention and *individual* therapy.

The Reproduction of Alienation

A main characteristic of developed capitalist societies is an increasing
division of labor, both in the production and legitimation spheres, with
the consequent separation of powers between governors and the
governed, administrators and the administrated, experts and laymen, and
intellectual and manual workers. Similarly, bourgeois medicine assumes a
division of labor in which the citizens are supposed to be the recipients of
care and the experts are supposed to be the providers and administrators
of therapy. The expropriation of political power from the citizenry that
takes place in the political process, and the absence of control over the
product and nature of work that workers face in the process of
production, are accompanied by the expropriation of control from the
patient and potential patient over the nature and definition of health in
the medical sector. And it is the bureaucracy—the medical profession—
that is supposed to administer and remove the mass of disease. In this
respect, the medical profession is assigned an impossible task, i.e. to solve
something that because of its actual economic and political nature, is
beyond its control. From the health maintenance point of view, then, the
medical care system is failing. And there is no way around that. But the
failure of medicine from this point of view does not mean that it is not
useful. To the contrary, the social utility of medicine is measured primarily in the arena of legitimation. Medicine is indeed socially useful to
the degree that the majority of people believe and accept the proposition
that what are actually politically caused conditions can be individually
solved by medical intervention. From the point of view of the capitalist
system, this is the actual utility of medicine—it contributes to the
legitimation of capitalism. And it is because of this legitimation function
that the medical profession is serving the interests of the capitalist system
and of the capitalist class.

The second point that merits attention is that the expropriation of political power, work, and health takes place not only individually, but collectively, i.e. expropriation is imposed on the collectivity of citizens. And it is the collective nature of that expropriation that requires not an individual, but a collective response. As we have seen, the aim of capitalist medicine is to reduce a collective phenomenon to an individual one. In this respect, and as I indicated before, far from conflicting with the ideology of medicine, the present self-care strategies are actually strengthening that ideology so long as they remain at the level of individual responses.

SECTION III:

THE MODE OF STATE INTERVENTION
IN THE HEALTH SECTOR

Mechanisms of State Intervention

Having discussed the nature, role, and characteristics of the state, let us now analyze the specific mechanisms of state intervention in capitalist societies. And let us begin by somewhat arbitrarily dividing those interventions into primarily two levels: one of negative and the other of positive selection.

A. Negative Selection Mechanisms

By negative selection, I mean that mode of intervention that systematically and continually excludes those strategies that conflict with the class nature of the capitalist society. This negative intervention takes place through (a) structural selective mechanisms, (b) ideological mechanisms, (c) decision-making mechanisms, and (d) repressive coercion mechanisms.[9]

Structural Selective Mechanisms. These mechanisms refer to the exclusion of alternatives that threaten the capitalist system, an exclusion that is inherent in the nature of the capitalist state. Offe mentions, for example, the constitutionally guaranteed right in all capitalist societies to private property, which excludes state conflict with that right and with the class

[9]In this article, I am using a modified version of Offe's categories. For a presentation of his theories of state intervention, see references 82–84. For a critique of Offe's work, see references 85–87.

nature that right determines. In fact, the overall priority given to property and capital accumulation explains why, when health and property conflict, the latter usually takes priority over the former. For example, the appalling lack of adequate legislation protecting the worker in most capitalist societies (including social democratic Sweden) contrasts most dramatically with the large array of laws protecting private property and its owners. The dramatic cuts in the already meager funds for federal occupational programs in the U.S. indicate that when a conflict appears between capital accumulation and property on the one hand and health on the other, the latter is, by definition, the loser (88). And the present outrage voiced by the French establishment when a factory owner was jailed for negligence shows that this "benign neglect" of workers, but strong concern for owners and property is not unique to the U.S.

This structural negative selective mechanism also appears in the implied assumption that all health programs and reforms have to take place within the set of class relations prevalent in capitalist societies. For example, in Britain, Bevan's Labour Party strategy of implementing the NHS (a victory for the British working class) assumed an unalterability of class relations in Britain. Indeed, the creation of the NHS was seen as taking place within the structure of capitalist Britain of 1948, respecting the class distribution of power both outside and within the health sector. Bevan relied very heavily on the consultants, who clearly were of upper class extraction and position, to break the general practitioner's resistance against the implementation of the NHS. As he proudly indicated, "I bought them with gold" (89). The strategy of using the nationalization of the health sector to break with the class structure outside and within the health sector, as Lenin did in the Soviet Union, was not even considered (90). Moreover, to reassure the medical profession in general and the consultants in particular, they were given dominant influence over the process of planning, regulation, and administration of the health sector (91). Actually, these mechanisms of class reassurance also operated in other nationalized sectors. As Coates has indicated, the men chosen by the Labour Government in the 1940s to lead the nationalized industries were all members of the managerial and ownership class of the former private industries (92). And as Shearer has indicated, the same has occurred in the U.S. (93). In summary, in all Western capitalist societies, nationalization has taken place within the set of class relations prevalent in those societies.

Ideological Mechanisms. These mechanisms insure the exclusion from the realm of debate of ideologies that conflict with the system. In other words, it is not only programs and policies, as indicated before, that are being automatically excluded, but, more importantly, conflicting ideologies as well. This is clearly shown in the lack of attention to and the lack of research in areas that conflict with the requirements and needs of the capitalist system. Reflecting the bourgeois bias of the medical research establishment for example, much priority is given to the assumedly individual causation of disease. One instance, among others, is that most research on heart disease—one of the main killers in society—has focused on diet, exercise, and genetic inheritance. On the study of these etiologies, millions of pounds, dollars, marks, and francs have been spent. However, in a fifteen-year study of aging, cited in a most interesting report prepared by a special task force to the Secretary of Health, Education, and Welfare in the U.S., it was found that the most important predictor of longevity was work satisfaction. Let me quote from that report:

> . . . the strongest predictor of longevity was work satisfaction. The second best predictor was over-all "happiness" . . . Other factors are undoubtedly important—diet, exercise, medical care, and genetic inheritance. But research findings suggest that these factors may account for only about 25% of the risk factors in heart disease, the major cause of death. That is, if cholesterol, blood pressure, smoking, glucose level, serum uric acid, and so forth, were perfectly controlled, only about one-fourth of coronary heart disease could be controlled. Although research on this problem has not led to conclusive answers, it appears that work role, work conditions, and other social factors may contribute heavily to this "unexplained" 75% of risk factors (94).

But very few studies have investigated these socio-political factors. Indeed, studies on such subjects as work satisfaction have a threatening potential to the actual controllers of the work process since, as Braverman has clearly shown, the nature of the capitalist process of production is what actually determines that alienating work (95). To change the former means to question the latter. In summary, the exclusion of ideologies which question or threaten the basic assumptions of the capitalist system is a most prevalent mechanism of state intervention, i.e. the exclusion as unthinkable of any alternatives to that system.

Decision Making Mechanisms. The decision making processes are heavily weighted in favor of certain groups and classes, and thus against certain others. For example, the mechanisms of selection and appointment of members to the new regional and area health planning and administrative agencies in Britain (96) and to the Health System Agencies in the U.S. (97) are conducive to the dominance over those bodies of individuals of the corporate and upper-middle classes, to the detriment of members of the lower-middle and working classes.

Repressive Coercion Mechanisms. The final form of negative selection, repressive coercion mechanisms, take place either through the use of direct force or, more importantly, by cutting (and thus nullifying) those programs that may conflict with sources of power within the state organism (e.g. the cutting of OEO in the U.S. because it developed into an alternative source of power to local government).

B. Positive Selection Mechanisms

By positive selection, I mean the type of state intervention that generates, stimulates, and determines a positive response favorable to overall capital accumulation, as opposed to a negative selection which excludes anticapitalist possibilities. Offe distinguishes between two types of such intervention—allocative and productive (98). In the former, the state regulates and coordinates the allocation of resources that have already been produced, while in the latter, the state becomes directly involved in the production of goods and services.

Allocative Intervention Policies. These policies are based on the authority of the state in influencing, guiding, and even directing the main activities of society, including the most important one—capital accumulation. The policies are put into effect primarily (although not exclusively) through laws that make certain behavior mandatory and through regulations that make certain claims legal. In the health sector, examples of the former are laws requiring doctors to register contagious disease with the state health department and for employers to install protective devices to prevent industrial accidents, while an example of the latter is regulations determining that certain categories of people receive health insurance. Both laws and regulations are determined and dictated in the world of politics. As Offe indicates, in allocative functions "policy and politics are not differentiated" (99). And, as such, those policies are determined by the different degrees of dominance of the branches of the state by pressure groups and factions primarily within the dominant class.

Here, we have to ask ourselves how we can go about studying those allocative policies and their class character? The most frequently used method is to analyze the ways, in either specific government policies or in historical events, that the different classes and their components relate *via interpersonal relationships* with the organs of the state and its intermediary institutions such as political parties, professional associations, etc.

Productive Intervention Policies. As I have indicated, productive intervention policies are those whereby the state directly participates in the production of resources, e.g. medical education in most Western capitalist countries, production of drugs in nationalized drug industries, management of public hospitals, medical research, etc. Before analyzing these activities, let me clarify a number of points that have an important bearing on the presentation of these productive activities.

- There is not always a clear-cut distinction between allocative and productive policies. Frequently health policies include elements of both. Most allocative functions are administered by the state apparatus, mainly the civil service or the administrative branch of the executive, while productive functions take place outside the administrative bodies of the state apparatus. For example, in the production of medical knowledge (research and teaching), the allocative functions are carried out by an administrative branch of the state apparatus, while their actual production is carried out by medical schools and research institutions that, although public institutions for the most part, are not directly run by the branch of the state apparatus in charge of the allocative function, nor by any other branch for that matter.

- Both allocative and productive policies have increased dramatically in all capitalist countries since World War II and, along with that increase, a shift has taken place from allocative to productive policies. An example of the latter is the production of medical knowledge, where there has been a shift in state intervention from an allocative function (e.g. subsidies, tax benefits) to actual production (e.g. nationalization of medical schools and research institutions). Similarly, there is a trend in the health sector to move from national insurance schemes (allocative) to national health services (productive). Britain in 1948, Quebec (Canada) in 1968, and Italy in the 1970s are each examples of that trend. In all capitalist countries, there has been an impressive growth of state intervention, primarily of the productive type of intervention, as measured by either public expenditures or public employment. Moreover, this growth has taken place mainly in the social (including health) services sector. In a recent survey of expenditures carried out by OECD among its member countries, for example, it is concluded that in all of them, public expenditures have grown and will continue to grow very dramatically, both proportionally and absolutely, during the period under study (1960–1980), and that the major characteristics of these changes are very substantial growth in (a) social services expenditures, including education, health and social security; (b) capital investments of an infrastructural character (e.g. roads); and (c) state aid to private industries (100). And in this growth of expenditures, the health sector occupies a prominent place. During the last twenty years, health expenditures in capitalist developed countries have grown faster than the GNP (101), and Table 1 presents the

Table 1

Health Expenditures as Percentage of GNP
in Several Western Capitalist Countries, 1950–1973

	1950	1960	1970	1973
England and Wales	4.1	3.9	4.9	5.3
United States	4.6	5.2	7.1	7.7
France	2.9	4.0	5.5	5.8
West Germany	—	4.5	—	—
Sweden	—	3.5	6.6	—

Source: reference 101.

percentage of the GNP represented by health expenditures in a sampling of these countries. Similarly, in terms of employment, the social services sector (including health) has been the fastest growing. Having described that growth, let me now analyze its nature and consequences.

The Reasons for the Growth of State Intervention

The growth of the health sector in developed capitalist countries is due to the growth of social needs, which are determined by the process of capital accumulation and by the heightening of the level of class struggle. Let me expand on each.

The Growth of Social Needs as Demanded
by the Process of Capital Accumulation

As indicated before, the primary role of state intervention is to facilitate the process of capital accumulation, i.e. to stimulate and strengthen the economy. Let us now discuss the main characteristics of that process of capital accumulation and analyze the sets of requirements from the different agencies of the state that are determined by that process. And a primary characteristic of that process of accumulation is, as indicated earlier, its concentration. Indeed, insurance, banking, manufacturing, and other sectors of economic life are in the hands of an increasingly small number of corporations that, for the most part, control the market in each sector (103). The consequences of that concentration are many but, among them, the most important is the type of technology and industrial development determined by and intended primarily to serve the needs of that concentration. And determined by that economic concentration and by that type of technological and industrial development are the following:

- *A division of labor, with a continuous demand for specialization* that fragments the process of production and ultimately the producer himself. And this specialization demands great involvement and investment from the state in order to guarantee the reproduction of labor needed for the system. Similarly in the health sector, the state allocates and produces the human resources needed for the delivery of health care, stimulating an increased specialization of labor necessary to sustain and legitimize the growing concentration, industrialization and hierarchicalization of that sector. In summary, and as expressed in Figure 1, increased economic concentration determines a growing concentration of political power and a greater need for state intervention to facilitate the type of industrialization demanded by that economic concentration—an industrialization that influences and determines the type of specialized medicine that is prevalent today.

Figure 1

The Dialectical Relationship between Concentration of
Economic Power and Industrialization of Society (Including Medicine)

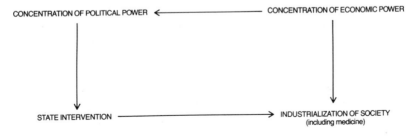

Let me clarify here that I believe the relationship among these categories to be dialectical, not linear, with a pattern of dominance that is expressed by the main direction of the arrow in Figure 1.

- *An invasion of all sectors of economic life by corporate capital.* Indeed, it is a tendency of the process of capital accumulation that the search for profits invades all sectors of economic life, including social services such as health (104), education (105), transportation (106), etc., etc. As Mandel has indicated:

> The logic of late capitalism is . . . to convert idle capital into service capital and simultaneously to replace service capital with productive capital, in other words, services with commodities; transport services with private cars; theatre and film services with private television sets; tomorrow, television programmes and educational instruction with video-cassettes (107).

In summary, it is the tendency of contemporary capitalism to convert public services into commodities to be bought and sold on the private market. Reflecting that tendency is the push by both conservatives in the U.K. and conservatives and large numbers of liberals in the U.S. to shift the delivery of health services back to the private sector (supposedly to enable them to be run more efficiently and more profitably) and to keep them there. And in this scheme, the payment for services is public, while the appropriation of profit is private. In brief, the state sector is footing the bill for the profit of capital.

- *An invasion of the spheres of social life by corporate capital and its process of industrialization,* causing dislocation, diswelfare, and insecurity that state intervention, through social services (including medicine) is in turn supposed to mitigate. The most important example, of course, is the alienation that the industrialized process of production causes in the working population—an alienation that becomes reflected in psychosomatic conditions which medicine is supposed to care for and cure. Similarly, occupational diseases and environmental damage are, for the most part, also corporately caused, but, according to bourgeois ideology, individually cured through medical intervention. In summary, the concentration of economic activities and its consequent process of industrialization create a process of diswelfare that, in turn, determines and requires the growth of state services.

- *An invasion of corporate capital into the spheres of private life,* with the commodification of all processes of interpersonal relationships, from sex to the pursuit of happiness. Indeed, according to corporate ideology, happiness depends on the amount and type of consumption, i.e. on what the citizen has, not on what he or she does.

- *An increased proletarianization of the population,* including the medical profession. As a result, the health professions have shifted from being independent entrepreneurs to becoming employees of private medical corporations (as in the U.S.) or employees of the state (as in the majority of European capitalist countries). In both cases, that process of proletarianization is stimulated by the state, with the assistance of the corporate segments of the capitalist class (108).

- *An increased concentration of resources in urban areas,* and deployment of resources to those areas, required and needed for the realization of capital. This process of urbanization necessitates a growth in the allocative functions of the state (e.g. land use legislation and city planning) and of productive functions (e.g. roads and sanitation) so as to support, guide, and direct that process in a way that is responsive to the needs of capital accumulation. It is worth underlining in this context that the majority of infrastructural services are consumed by components of Capital and not by private households. For example, three-quarters of the U.S. water supply is consumed by industry and agriculture (mainly corporate), while private households consume less than one-quarter. Water supply, however, is paid for largely from funds coming from the latter, not from the former (109).

In summary, then, the economic concentration typical of the present stage of capitalism—usually referred to as monopoly capitalism—determines (a) an invasion by corporate capital of all spheres of economic, social and even private life in its quest for profits, and (b) a specific type of technological development and industrialization (both of which processes are summarized in Figure 2) that requires increased state intervention to stimulate and facilitate that concentration, as well as to rectify the dislocation of general well being created by that concentration.

Moreover, this process of economic concentration and its concomitant industrialization determines a model of production and distribution in medicine that replicates the characteristics of the overall process of economic production and distribution, i.e. specialization, concentration, urbanization and a technical orientation of medicine. The nature of medicine, then, and its relation to the overall process of production determine in large degree its *characteristics.* And its position within that

Figure 2
The Dialectical Relationship between Society and Medicine

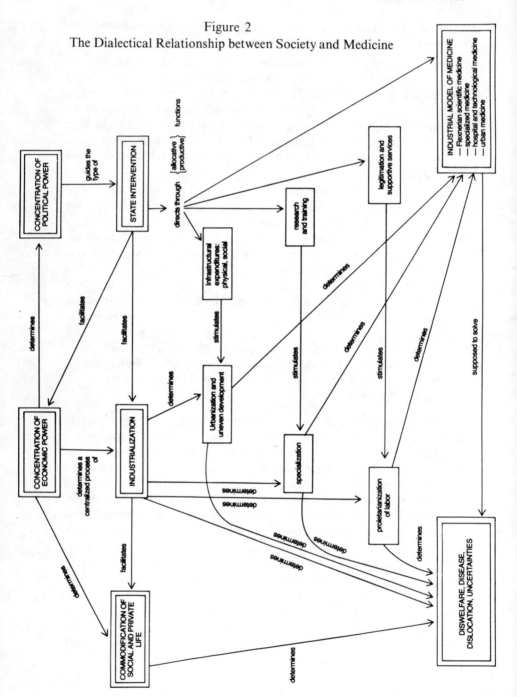

process of production explains its function, which is to take care of and solve the unsolvable—the diswelfare and dysfunctions created by that very process of production.

The Level of Class Struggle

The tendencies explained in the previous section are the result of the growing needs of capital accumulation which take place within the context of a continuous conflict between Capital and Labor—a conflict primarily between the capitalist class and the working class. Indeed, the working class aims continuously at extracting significant concessions from the state, over and above what the state considers sufficient for the needs of capital accumulation defined in the previous section. For example, it is impossible to understand the creation of the NHS in Britain without taking into account the relationship of class forces in Britain and the wartime radicalization of the working class that had called into question "the survival of capitalism." As Forsyth has indicated:

> Rightly or wrongly the British Government at the outbreak of war could not be sure that large sections of the working class were entirely satisfied about the reasons for fighting the war . . . For the sake of public morale the Government tried to make it clear that after the war things were going to be very different from the heartbreak conditions of the "thirties" (110).

The much heralded consensus on the need for a national health service that existed among Labour and Conservative politicians was the result of the radicalization of the working class on the one hand, and the concern for the survival of capitalism by the capitalist class and the state on the other.[10] Indeed, labor movements have historically viewed social services (including health) as part of the *social wage,* to be defended and increased in the same way that *money wages* are. In fact, Wilensky has shown how the size of social wages depends, in large degree, on the level of militancy of the labor movements (111). Thus, contrary to popular belief, the size and nature of social benefits in terms of social services is higher in France and Italy than in Scandinavia or even in Britain. And I attribute this to the greater militancy of the unions in those countries and to the existence of mass Socialist and Communist parties (whose platforms are, at least in theory, anticapitalist) that force an increase of social wages upon the

[10] While that radicalization triggered the creation of the NHS, the implementation of that legislation was skewed to favor and replicate the class structure and hierarchicalization of labor prevalent then as today. Indeed, the concession by the capitalist class and victory of the working class could not conflict, or conflict as little as possible, with either the class structure of Britain, or with the process of capital accumulation that determined it.

state. Another indicator is the percentage of GNP spent on social security which, in 1965, was 17.5 per cent in Italy, 18.3 per cent in France, but only 7.9 per cent in the U.S. (112). The practical absence of a comprehensive coverage for social benefits in the U.S. is also undoubtedly due to the lack of an organized left party.

Thus, in the Labor-Capital conflict, the labor movement demands (a) an increase of social wages, the comprehensiveness and level of which depend on the strength of working class pressure; (b) an increase in jobs to counteract the tendency toward unemployment characteristic of contemporary capitalism. In that respect, the large increase in public employment, for example—particularly at the provincial, state or local government levels—is in no small degree due to the demand for the state to absorb the surplus population; (c) provision of services, such as welfare, social security, and unemployment insurance to smooth down and cushion the dislocation, uncertainty and diswelfare created by the process of capital accumulation; (d) an increased demand by labor to control the process of production through workers' control;[11] and (e) a demand for public ownership of the means of production, which has meant that even governing social democratic parties are forced to pay lip service to that objective.[12]

In summary, then, the nature and growth of the state in contemporary capitalist societies can be attributed to the increased *social needs of capital* and *social demands of labor*. And in order to understand the nature of any state policy, including health policy, we have to place our analysis within those parameters. Having said that, let me clarify two points. First, there is no single-factor explanation of social policy. Rather, it is explained by the combination of factors already mentioned. And the nature and number of those combinations will depend on the *historical* origins of each factor, the *political* form determining the factor and its relation to others, and its *function* in that specific social formation. Second, there is no clear cut dichotomy between the social needs of

[11]It is worth underlining that the demand for workers' control—different from workers' participation—has arisen in most Western capitalist societies from the base and not the top of the labor movement. For an interesting account of the evolution of workers' demands to control the process of work in Italy, see reference 113.

[12]See, for example, Clause 4 of the *Governing Constitution of the British Labour Party,* which reads that the primary aim of the Party is "to secure for the workers by hand or by brain the full fruits of their industry and the most equitable distribution thereof that may be possible, upon the basis of the common ownership of the means of production, distribution and exchange, and the best obtainable system of popular administration and control of each industry or service."

capital and the social demands of labor. Any given policy can serve both. Indeed, social policies that serve the interests of the working class can be subsequently adapted to benefit the interests of the dominant class. As Miliband and others have shown so well, the "bias of the system" has always insured that these policies can be deflected to suit the capitalist class. Indeed, history shows that concessions won by labor in the class struggle become, *in the absence of further struggle,* modified to serve the interests of the capitalist class.

The Present Fiscal Crisis of the State: A Final Note on the Health Sector in Contemporary Capitalist Societies

I end this article, then, by underlining once again the two main characteristics of contemporary capitalism, i.e. the concentration of capital and the consequent growth of the state. In this scenario, the growth of the state (and the growth of medicine within it) is both a product and a cause of the expansion of monopoly capital. In Marxist terms, the growing socialization of production necessitates greater state intervention to insure private capital accumulation and profitability. But this growth of state intervention and state expenditure requires raising ever-increasing revenues that are forever insufficient to pay for them. Thus, the continuous fiscal crisis of the state (114).

The main characteristics of the state's response to this crisis have been (a) a cutting of social wages, (b) an increasing demand for planning of the economy, which requires still further centralization of power in contemporary capitalism, and (c) a growing demand for rationalization of the system, with calls for higher productivity and efficiency.

These three characteristics of state response to its fiscal crises are also reflected in the situation of the medical sector in capitalist societies. This reality is typified, first, by cuts in health expenditures resulting from the determination of the capitalist class to "save the economy" at whatever cost and put first and foremost the need for private capital accumulation. As a result, a political struggle is taking place over the state's goal to cut social wages and, in particular, to cut those portions such as medical care, care of the elderly, and welfare services which are considered by capital as contributing least to the productivity of the system. And in all these societies, the argument put forward in defense of such cuts is the need to shift capital from unproductive to productive sectors in order to increase private capital accumulation. Consequently, these cuts in health and social services have been accompanied by increased assistance to private industry. Needless to say, the working class (although not always its leaders) has resisted these cuts, considering social wages as a needed complement to their money wages. One instance, among others, of this resistance is the strike of coal miners in Yorkshire in order to protest the cuts in the NHS and support a rise in pay for nurses.

Second, there is increasing centralization by the state (and primarily by the executive branch and its administrative apparatus) of the direction of social and health policy. Examples of this centralization are the reorganization of the NHS in Great Britain and of the health planning apparatus in the U.S. This centralization manifests itself in (a) the creation of regional and local bodies (e.g. Health System Agencies in the U.S. and Area Health Authorities in Britain) that bypass local government and are ultimately accountable to the central government; and (b) a shift of power from the legislative to the executive branch of government, with an increasing allocation of decision-making power to agencies of the state apparatus (e.g. major decisions in the U.S. health sector are increasingly made by the Office of Management and the Budget of the White House).

Finally, the increased demand for rationalization of the system forces the central government to develop both mechanisms of cost control and alternative ways of organizing the delivery system (e.g. emphasis on primary care) and different types of personnel (e.g. nurse practitioners) that can do the job "cheaper." In all these reforms, a primary motive is the reduction of costs. Underlying these changes, there are ideological changes as well, with both an increasing focus on modifying individual behavior as the best payoff for improving health and a growing skepticism concerning the effectiveness of medical intervention.

These, then, are the main characteristics of the medical sector in Western capitalist societies today, and they are determined by the historical, political and functional factors discussed in the course of this article.

In summary, I have aimed to show that if we are to understand the nature, composition, distribution and function of the medical care sector in Western developed capitalist societies, we must first understand the distribution of power in those societies and the nature, role, and instrumentality of the state. This understanding leads us to realize that (a) the assumedly transcended and diluted category of social class is a much needed category in understanding the distribution of power in our societies; and that (b) class struggle, far from being an outmoded concept of interest only to "vulgar" Marxists, is most relevant indeed and as much needed today to understand the nature of our societies and of our health sectors as it was when Marx and Engels wrote that "class struggle is the motor of history."

Needless to say, this interpretation is a minority voice in our Western academic setting. It is in conflict with the prevalent explanations of the health sector, and this accounts for its exclusion from the realm of debate. Still, its veracity will be affirmed not by its "popularity" in the corridors of power, which will be nil, but in its verification on the terrain of history. It is because of this that I dedicated this article to all those with whom I share a praxis aimed at building up a society of truly free and self-governing men and women—a society in which, as Marx indicated, the state (and I would add medicine) will be converted "from an organ superimposed upon society into one completely subordinated to it" (115).

References

1. Cochrane, A.L. *Effectiveness and Efficiency: Random Reflections on Health Services.* Nuffield Provincial Hospitals Trust, London, 1972, p. 70.

2. Titmuss, R. *Commitment to Welfare.* Unwin University Books, London, 1968.

3. Tudor Hart, J. The inverse care law. *Lancet* 1 (7696): 405–412, 1971.

4. For an answer to and critique of Cochrane's dismissal of class inequities of consumption, see Tudor Hart, J. An assault on all custom. *International Journal of Health Services* 3 (1): 101–104, 1973.

5. For a representative reference, see Bice, T.W., Eichhorn, R.L. and Fox, P.D. Socio-economic status and use of physician services: a reconsideration. *Medical Care* 10 (3): 261–271, 1972. For a critique of equalization of consumption by social class in the U.S., see Berki, S.E. Comments on "Socioeconomic status and use of physician services: a reconsideration." *Medical Care* 11 (3): 259, 1973.

6. Anderson, O. *Health Care: Can There Be Equity? The United States, Sweden, and England.* John Wiley and Sons, New York, 1972.

7. *Ibid.,* p. 26.

8. *Ibid.,* pp. 24–25.

9. Westergaard, J.H. Sociology: the myth of classlessness. In Blackburn, R. *Ideology in Social Science.* Fontana, New York, 1972, p. 121.

10. Habermas, J. *Toward a Rational Society: Student Protest, Science and Politics.* Beacon Press, Boston, 1971.

11. Marcuse, H. *One Dimensional Man.* Beacon Press, Boston, 1964.

12. Aronowitz, S. *False Promises: The Shaping of American Working-Class Consciousness.* McGraw Hill, New York, 1973.

13. Learmonth, A. Regional disparities in the health sector. *Health.* Open University Press, London, 1972.

14. Miliband, R. *The State in Capitalist Society.* Weidenfeld and Nicolson, London, 1970.

15. Poulantzas, N. *Political Power and Social Classes.* New Left Books, London, 1973.

16. Poulantzas, N. *Classes in Contemporary Capitalism.* New Left Books, London, 1975.

17. Anderson, O. *op. cit.,* p. 28. It is worth indicating that Anderson, along with many others in political sociology literature, seems to confuse the government with the state. Indeed, the functions listed by Anderson as functions of the government (p. 29) are actually the functions of the state. The executive and legislative branches of the state (the government) are only part of the overall structure of the state. For a further expansion of this point, see: The state system and the state elite. In Miliband, R. *op. cit.,* p. 49.

18. There are many authors who uphold variants of this theory. The most representative is Dahl, R.A. *A Preface to Democratic Theory.* University of Chicago Press, Chicago, 1956. In medical care literature, the most representative is Anderson, O. *op. cit.,* whose inheritance from Dahl is acknowledged, and Fuchs, V. *Who Shall Live: Health, Economics and Social Choice.* Basic Books, New York, 1975.

19. Hart Poll results reported in Bender, M. Will the bicentennial see the death of free enterprise? *New York Times,* Jan., 4, 1976, p. 27.

20. Representative of this analysis in the United States are the most informative volumes by Alford, R. *Health Care Politics.* University of Chicago Press, Chicago, 1975, and Marmor, T. *The Politics of Medicare.* Aldine Publishing Co., Chicago, 1973. In the United Kingdom, representatives are Willcocks, J. *The Creation of the National Health Service. A Study of Pressure Groups and a Major Social Policy Decision.* Routledge and Kegan Paul, London, 1967, and Eckstein, H. *The English Health Service: Its Origins, Structure and Achievement.* Harvard University Press, Cambridge, MA., 1958.

21. For a further explanation of the rationality of capitalism, see Godelier, M. *Rationality and Irrationality in Economics.* Monthly Review Press, New York, 1973.

22. For an expanded critique of power elite theories, see Poulantzas, N. The problems of the capitalist state. *New Left Review* 58, 1969, and Economic elites and dominant class, in Miliband, R. *op. cit.,* p. 23.

23. Illich, I. *Medical Nemesis: The Expropriation of Health.* Calder and Boyars, London, 1975. Also, a similar paradigm is presented in Freidson, E. *Doctoring Together: A Study of Professional Social Control.* Elsevier, New York, 1975.

24. Mahler, H. Health—a demystification of medical technology. *Lancet* 2 (7940): 829–833, 1975.

25. Navarro, V. The industrialization of fetishism or the fetishism of industrialization: a critique of Ivan Illich. *Social Science & Medicine* 9 (7): 351–363, 1975. (See also pp. 103–131 of this volume.)

26. Susser, M. Ethical components in the definition of health. *International Journal of Health Services* 4 (3): 539–548, 1974.

27. Miliband, R. *op. cit.*

28. Poulantzas, N. The problems of the capitalist state. *op. cit.* (reference 22).

29. See Miliband, R. Marx and the state. In Miliband, R. and Saville, J. (eds.) *The Socialist Register, 1965.* Merlin Press, London, 1966, p. 278.

30. Letter from Engels to Bloch, September 21, 1890. In Marx, K. and Engels, F. *Selected Correspondence,* Moscow, 1963, p. 498.

31. Marx, K. *The Eighteenth Brumaire of Louis Bonaparte.* International Publishers, New York, 1969, p. 15.

32. Introduction. In Navarro, V. *The Political Economy of Social Security and Medical Care in the USSR* (in process).

33. Althusser, L. and Balibar, E. *Reading Capital.* Pantheon Books, New York, 1970.

34. Godelier, M. *op. cit.*

35. Poulantzas, N. *Political Power and Social Classes.*

36. The best reference on structuralism in the health sector is the excellent article by Renaud, M. On the structural constraints to state intervention in health. *International Journal of Health Services* 5 (4): 559–571, 1975. Also, Polack, J.C. *La Medecine du Capital.* Maspero, Paris, 1970.

37. Gates, F. Capital and labor. Undated Memorandum, Gates Collection, Rockefeller Foundation Archives.

38. Glyn, A. and Sutcliffe, B. *British Capitalism. Workers and the Profit Squeeze.* Penguin Books, Middlesex, 1972.

39. Miliband, R. Reply to N. Poulantzas. *New Left Review* 59, 1970.

40. Miliband, R. Poulantzas and the capitalist state. *New Left Review* 82, 1973.

41. Laclau, E. Poulantzas-Miliband debate. *Economy and Society* 4 (1), 1975.

42. One of the most informative and instructive discussions of the nature of corporate state theories is O'Connor, J. *The Corporations and the State.* Harper Books, New York, 1974. Also, by the same author, *The Fiscal Crisis of the State.* St. Martin's Press, New York, 1973. For a French version of corporate statism, see Herzog, P. *Politique Economique.* Maspero, Paris, 1971.

43. Marx, K. and Engels, F. *The Communist Manifesto.* International Publishers, New York, 1960.

44. Gough, I. Review of "The Fiscal Crisis of the State." *Bulletin of the Conference of Socialist Economists* 4 (1): 823, 1975.

45. Miliband, R. *The State in Capitalist Society,* p. 11.

46. Offe, C. The theory of the capitalist state and the problem of policy formation. In Lindberg, L. et al. (eds.). *Stress and Contradiction in Modern Capitalism.* Lexington Books, London, 1975, p.126.

47. Sigerist, H.E. *Landmarks in the History of Hygiene.* Oxford University Press, London, 1956.

48. Quoted in George, V. and Wilding, P. Social values, social class and social policy. *Social and Economic Administration* 6 (3): 236–248, 1972.

49. Offe, C. *op. cit.,* p. 127.

50. For an analysis of businessmen predominant in the governmental corridors of power in the U.S. and the U.K., see Lasswell, H.D. et al. *The Comparative Study of Elites.* Stanford University Press, Stanford, CA., 1952; Mills, C.W. *The Power Elite.* Oxford University Press, New York, 1956; and Guttsman, W.L. *The British Political Elite.* MacGibbon and Kee, London, 1963.

51. Kilborn, P.K. Britain slashes spending on social-welfare items. *New York Times,* February 21, 1976.

52. The budget: a special analysis. Special issue of *National Journal* 8 (5), 1976.

53. For an analysis of the increased reliance of state expenditure on credit, see: Permanent inflation. In Mandel, E. *Late Capitalism.* New Left Books, London, 1975, pp. 409–437.

54. Offe, C. *op. cit.,* p. 126.

55. Coates, D. *The Labour Party and the Struggle for Socialism.* Cambridge University Press, London and New York, 1975, p. 68.

56. Domhoff, G.W. *The Higher Circles: The Governing Class in America.* Vintage Books, New York, 1971.

57. Miliband, R. *The State in Capitalist Society.*

58. Tudor Hart, J. Industry and the health services. *Lancet* 2 (7829): 611, 1973.

59. Navarro, V. The political economy of medical care; an explanation of the composition, nature and functions of the present health sector of the United States. *International Journal of Health Services* 5 (1):65–94, 1975. (See also pp. 135–169 of this volume.)

60. Mandel, E. *op. cit.,* p. 492.

61. This debate is reproduced in Blackburn, R. *op. cit.,* pp. 239–262.

62. Thorborn, G. Power in the kingdom of Sweden. *International Socialist Journal* 2 (59): 490–494, 1965.

63. See Democratic Junta and Convergencia Democratic programs for the support of Marxist parties to the democratization of Spain. *Cambio,* January, 1976.

64. Mandel, E. *op. cit.,* p. 494.

65. Applebaum, A. New York City hospitals; the financial crunch. *Hospitals* 50 (2): 59, 1975.

66. For a critique of the market ideologies in the health sector, see Navarro, V. National health insurance and the strategy for change. *Milbank Memorial Fund Quarterly / Health and Society,* 51 (2):223–251, 1973.

67. Revised list of NHI advisory panel members issued. *Washington Information: National Health Insurance* 2–5, 1975.

68. Cambridge Survey Polls. *Health Security News,* 1976.

69. Complete Hart Polls. In *Common Sense,* September 1, 1975, pp. 16–17. Also quoted in Bender, M. Will the bicentennial see the death of free enterprise? *op. cit.*

70. For an expansion of the political consequence of economic concentration, see Gough, I. State expenditure in advanced capitalism. *New Left Review* 92: 53–92, 1975.

71. Lenin, V. *The State and Revolution.* International Publishers, New York, 1932.

72. Trilateral Commission. *Governability of Democracies. Report of the Trilateral Task Force.* New York, 1975. For an excellent critique of this report, see Wolfe, A. Capitalism shows its force. *Nation* 221 (18): 557–563, 1975.

73. Wolfe, A. New directions in the marxist theory of politics. *Politics & Society* 4 (2): 149, 1974.

74. Miller, A. H. Political issues and trust in Government: 1964–1970. *American Political Science Review* 68, 1974.

75. Gramsci, A. *Prison Notebooks.* International Publishers, New York, 1971.

76. Navarro, V. The industrialization of fetishism or the fetishism of industrialization. *op. cit.*

77. For an excellent analysis of this point, see Braverman, H. *Labor and Monopoly Capital.* Monthly Review Press, New York, 1975.

78. McKeown, T. A historical appraisal of the medical task. In McKeown, T. (ed.). *Medical History and Medical Care; A Symposium of Perspectives.* Oxford University Press, New York and London, 1971, p. 29.

79. See the excellent description by Engels of the conditions among the English working class for a view of the effect of nascent capitalism on the health of the population. Engels, F. *The Condition of the Working Class in England.* Stanford University Press, Stanford, CA., 1958.

80. For further discussion, see Navarro, V. The underdevelopment of health of working America: causes, consequences and possible solutions. *American Journal of Public Health* 66 (6): 538–547 1976. (See also pp. 82–99 of this volume.)

81. See, among other examples, Lalonde, M. *A New Perspective on the Health of Canadians: A Working Document.* Government Printing Office, Government of Canada, 1975.

82. Offe, C. Political authority and class structures—an analysis of state capitalist societies. *International Journal of Sociology* 2 (1): 73–108, 1972.

83. Offe, C. The abolition of market control and the problem of legitimacy. *Kapitalistate* 1: 109, 1973.

84. Offe, C. and Ronge, V. Theses on the theory of the state. *New German Critique* 6: 137, 1975.

85. Biermann, S.S., Christiansen, V. and Dohse, K. Class domination and the political system: a critical interpretation of recent contributions by Claus Offe. *Kapitalistate* 2:60, 1973.

86. Rusconi, G. Marxism in West Germany, *Telos* 25, 1975.

87. Muller, W. and Neususs, C. The illusion of state socialism. *Telos* 25, 1975.

88. See the present cuts in OSHA, where the rationale is that they are too expensive and that they interfere with the process of capital accumulation. Burnham, D. Ford termed cool to 3 key agencies. *New York Times,* January 16, 1976, p. 1.

89. See Tudor Hart, J. Primary care in the industrial areas of Britain: evolution and current problems. *International Journal of Health Services* 2 (3): 349–365, 1972, and Bevan and the Doctors. *Lancet* 2 (7839): 1196–1197, 1973.

90. For Lenin's strategy in health services, see Leninism and medicine. In Navarro, V. *The Political Economy of Social Security and Medical Care in the USSR. op. cit.*

91. For an excellent analysis of the professional dominance in the NHS, see Robson, J. The NHS company inc. ? the social consequence of the professional dominance in the National Health Service. *International Journal of Health Services* 3 (3): 413–426, 1973. Also Draper, P. and Smart, T. Social science and health policy in the United Kingdom: some contributions of the social sciences to the bureaucratization of the National Health Service. *International Journal of Health Services* 4 (3): 453–470, 1974.

92. Coates, D. *The Labour Party and the Struggle for Socialism.* Cambridge University Press, London and New York, 1975, p. 48.

93. Shearer, D. The salt of public enterprise. *Nation,* February 21, 1976.

94. Special Task Force to the Secretary of Health, Education, and Welfare. *Work in America.* M.I.T. Press, Cambridge, MA., 1973, pp. 77–79.

95. Braverman, H. *op. cit.*

96. Tudor Hart, J. Industry and the health service. *Lancet* 2 (7829): 611, 1973.

97. Navarro, V. The political economy of medical care. *International Journal of Health Services* 5 (1): 65–93, 1975.

98. Offe, C. The theory of the capitalist state. *op. cit.,* p. 128.

99. *Ibid.*

100. OECD, *Expenditure Trends in OECD Countries, 1960–1980.* Mentioned in Gough, I. *op. cit.,* pp. 61–62.

101. Maxwell, R. *Health Care, The Growing Dilemma: Needs Versus Resources in Western Europe, the U. S. and the USSR.* McKinsey and Company, New York, 1975, p. 18.

102. *Ibid.,* p. 102.

103. See Sweezy, P. and Baran, P. *Monopoly Capital.* Monthly Review Press, New York, 1966.

104. For the increased dominance of financial capital in the funding of medical care in the U.S., see Navarro, V. The political economy of medical care. *op. cit.*

105. Bowles, S. and Gintis, H. *Schooling in Capitalist America: Educational Reform and the Contradictions of Economic Life.* Basic Books, New York, 1976.

106. Yago, G. *State Policy, Corporate Planning and Transportation Needs,* University of Wisconsin, Madison, 1974 (mimeographed).

107. Mandel, E. *op. cit.,* p. 406.

108. Editorial, Doctors and the State. *Wall Street Journal,* January 16, 1976.

109. O'Connor, J. *The Fiscal Crisis of the State. op. cit.,* p. 175.

110. Forsyth, G. *Doctors and State Medicine: A Study of the British Health Service.* Pitman and Sons, London, 1973, p. 16.

111. Wilensky, H.L. *The Welfare State and Equality.* University of California Press, Berkeley and Los Angeles, 1975.

112. International Labor Organization. *The Cost of Social Security, 1964–66.* Geneva, 1972, pp. 317–323.

113. Proctor, J. and Proctor, R. Capitalist development: class struggle and crisis in Italy, 1945–1975. *Monthly Review* 27:21–36, 1976.

114. For an excellent elaboration of this point, see O'Connor, J. *The Fiscal Crisis of the State.*

115. Marx, K. *Critique of the Gotha Program.* International Publishers, New York, 1938.

ACKNOWLEDGMENTS: We should like to express our sincere appreciation to the following sources for permission to reprint articles in this current volume:

"The Political and Economic Origins of the Underdevelopment of Health in Latin America"

Based on a presentation at the Pan American Conference on Health Manpower Planning held in Ottowa, September 10-14, 1973.

Awarded the 1974 John Kosa Memorial Prize.

Subsequently published under the title "The Underdevelopment of Health or the Health of Underdevelopment: An Analysis of the Distribution of Human Health Resources in Latin America" in *Politics and Society* 4(2): 267-293, 1974 and in the *International Journal of Health Services* 4(1): 5-27, 1974.

"Allende's Chile: A Case Study in the Breaking with Underdevelopment"

Based on a presentation at the International Health Seminar held at Harvard University, February 1974.

Subsequently published under the title "What Does Chile Mean: An Analysis of Events in the Health Sector Before, During and After Allende's Administration" in *The Milbank Memorial Fund Quarterly, Health and Society* 52(2): 93-130, 1974.

"Health and Medicine in the Rural United States: Its Political and Economic Determinants"

Based on a presentation at the First National Conference on Rural America in Washington, D.C., April 14-17, 1975.

Subsequently published in *Inquiry* 13(2):111–121, 1976. © 1976 Blue Cross Association.

"The Underdevelopment of Health of Working America: Causes, Consequences, and Possible Solutions"

Based on a presentation in the 103rd Annual Meeting of the American Public Health Association on the theme "Health and Work in America," held in Chicago, November 1975.

Subsequently appeared in the *American Journal of Public Health* 66(6):538–547, 1976.

"The Industrialization of Fetishism: A Critique of Ivan Illich"

Modified version published under the title "The Industrialization of Fetishism or the Fetishism of Industrialization: A Critique of Ivan Illich" in *Social Science and Medicine* 9: 351-363, 1975 and in the *International Journal of Health Services* 5(3): 351-371, 1975.

"An Explanation of the Composition, Nature, and Functions of the Present Health Sector of the United States"

Based on a presentation at the Annual Conference of the New York Academy of Medicine, April 25-26, 1974.

Modified versions appeared under the title "Social Policy Issues: An Explanation of the Composition, Nature and Functions of the Present Health Sector of the United States" in the *Bulletin of the New York Academy of Medicine* 51(1): 199-234, 1975 and in the *International Journal of Health Services* 5(1): 65-94, 1975.

"The Labor Force: Women as Producers of Services in the Health Sector of the United States"

Modified version presented at the International Conference on Women in Health, sponsored by the Health Resources Administration of the Department of Health, Education, and Welfare and held in Washington, D.C., June 16-18, 1975.

"Social Class, Political Power, and the State: Their Implications in Medicine"

Based on a presentation at the Colloque International de Sociologie Medicale held in Paris in July 1976.

Library of Congress Cataloging in Publication Data

Navarro, Vicente.
   Medicine under capitalism.

   Bibliography: p.
   1. Medical economics. 2. Medical care--United
States. 3. Medical care--Latin America. I. Title.
RA410.5.N33   362.1'09181'2   76-28521
ISBN 0-88202-116-8